IT'S NOT ABOUT YOU!

a mother and daughter's journey

Cindy Daniel
and
Robin Cieszinski

with Nancee Biank, MSW, LCSW

IT'S NOT ABOUT YOU!
a mother and daughter's journey
Published by Batelier Publishing
Printed in the United States of America
Copyright © Cindy Daniel 2006

Teens and Cancer in the Family
Copyright © Nancee Biank 2006
Published by permission

Amazon.com book reviews
published by permission
Copyright © Amazon.com

All Rights Reserved
ISBN-13:978-0-9789429-2-2
ISBN-10:0-9789429-2-2

Excerpt from Re-labelling Guilt; an article by Alison McWalter, *Alberta Caregivers Association-Bi-Weekly eNews,* 2004 published by permission.

Cover art by Erica Well

Acknowledgments

To Megan, Ana, Dana, Laura, Sarah, Lauren and Lindsay — for sharing their stories.

To Nancee Biank, Alison McWalter, and Kathy Kompare — for their professional contributions.

To Gayle Newkirk, Sherri Posey, and Carrie Wilson — for their encouragement and unfailing friendship.

To Lonnie Cruse — for constructive criticism and gentle editing.

To Erica Well — for capturing the mood.

To Ernest and Billye Godwin — for paving our road with love and faith.

And, to our husbands, Jeff & Mike — for their unconditional love.

                    -- *Cindy & Robin*
                       October 2006

Thank you, Matt,
for being strong
when we needed you...

IT'S NOT ABOUT YOU!

a mother and daughter's journey

Foreword

Foreword

This book WON'T give you all the answers. We don't have them. However, this book WILL tell you what we went through, how we handled it, and possibly teach someone—through our example—what NOT to do.

Ten years ago, when the doctor told me my mammogram was abnormal, I remember my family trying to reassure me, saying it was "probably nothing." At the time my response was, "I think it's more than *nothing*, but it's not more than I can *handle*." And, since I'm writing this story, you can tell I've managed to handle it so far.

However, this story is not about me. It's about my daughter Robin, who has spent the past ten years battling fear and anxiety, it's about all the teenage girls who suffer in silence as they watch and worry if their moms will be around next year, and it's about the mothers who have their breasts removed *and* their daughters' well-being destroyed by this incurable disease.

One out of every eight women is diagnosed with breast cancer. And I guarantee you, one of the first concerns she will have is how to tell her family. Should she act strong, downplay the seriousness to keep her loved ones from worrying? Or, should she show them her fear, her vulnerability, so they can draw strength from one another? Will she turn to God for hope or blame Him for her illness?

I can't tell you the right way to break the news to your daughter, son, husband, or parents. And, honestly, I don't know if there is ONE correct answer for everyone. But I DO know that I didn't get it right.

Ten years ago, I was diagnosed with cancer and my daughter's life would never be the same.

IT'S ABOUT THE MOMENT OF TRUTH

The diagnosis

I'm going to start the book by talking about how this experience affected ME, because I think you need to know some of the backstory, to better understand how we got so screwed up. The pressures I put on Robin and the things she went through in the beginning are all a part of the big picture.

Oh sure, she was a hormonal fifteen-year-old, so how do I really know where things got crazy? I don't. But I'm pretty sure it started somewhere around the time I was diagnosed.

Around Chapter Two Robin will start jumping in a lot with her feelings and thoughts. In fact, you may probably start identifying with her right away. Which may or may not be a good thing. Robin's words will be shown in 'bold italics' so you'll be able to tell *when she's talking.*

Nancy Biank, a psychologist who specializes in helping children of all ages deal with cancer in a loved one, will contribute her professional opinion, comment on how Robin and I made it through our experience, and offer support and advice

Regardless, here we go. Starting where all stories start. At the beginning...

My family was lucky. We'd never had to face cancer. It was one of those terrible things that happened to everyone else, but not us. So when I started having abnormal things happening to my breast I didn't know the 'right way' to tell my kids, or even if there was a right way. At that point, I just had to trust my instincts. So I told the kids about my doctor appointments, keeping the tone light so as not to upset them. And, let's face it, kids don't really care to hear about their moms' breast problems anyway; it kind of went in one ear and out the other.

My son, Matt, seemed nonplussed. He was seventeen at the time, just a month away from his eighteenth birthday; the only thing he had on his mind was celebrating his manhood.

My daughter, Robin, was busy coping with the problems that all young girls have as soon as their hormones hit; mood swings, boys, and deciding whether or not they like their bodies, their friends, and their moms.

You should know that my cancer didn't show it itself in the normal manner. I never felt a lump in my breast. The only thing I noticed was a few clear drops of fluid from my nipple. My gynecologist told me that since it wasn't discolored or painful they advised to watch and see if it continued. But, again, this is where instincts came in—I knew something wasn't right. So I became proactive.

At my urging, the doctor ordered blood work to check my Prolactin level, to identify if there was a hormone factor making me lactate (produce milk.) However, the test came back 'normal,' meaning I wasn't lactating and there was no medical reason for my nipple discharge.

Although I was only thirty-five at the time, with no family history of breast cancer, I requested a mammogram. I wasn't in a high-risk group, but the doctor ordered one anyway, for my peace of mind. And, as the doctor suspected, the mammogram came back normal.

At first...

The following day the radiologist called and said he'd decided to take a second look at my films, at which time he saw a questionable area. "It's probably not anything to worry about," he said. "It looks like an inflammation in the ducts. Maybe an infection."

And the journey began.

My mom's journey began at that point. But mine didn't start until later. I don't even remember ever being afraid for my mom in the beginning, because whatever she told me about her mammogram didn't worry me. I honestly don't even remember what she told me until she found out it was cancer.

The radiologist ordered a com-

pression mammogram, also referred
to as a 'spot compression.' Apply-
ing pressure to a smaller area of
tissue using a compression plate
or cone results in better tissue
separation and allows an enhanced
visualization of the area in question.

This procedure resulted in a
better view, showing a clearer
picture of what looked like in-
flamed duct glands in my left nipple.

Next, in order for the doctor
to better define the disease process, inflammation or perhaps infection, a ductogram was scheduled. The radiologist informed me
at this point that a consultation
with a general surgeon was also in
order; a surgeon being the one who
would construct a treatment plan.

I found a great surgeon who
specialized in diseases of the
breast. She scheduled the ductogram immediately and said, "I'm
ninety-nine percent sure it's going to be benign (not cancer,) but
I think we need to biopsy it to
make sure."

Now, for the sake of time, I
won't detail everything a ducto-

gram is like. Do a *Google* search for it on the Internet for more info. But the short version of the story is that they stick cannulas, which look like three-inch needles, directly into your nipple. Sounds a bit like medieval torture, doesn't it? They send a dye into the cannulas and watch through the x-ray equipment as the dye travels through the ducts in your breast to highlight any abnormalities.

Oh, and they squeeze your breast really, really hard before they do it to try to get it to leak so they know which duct to go in.

Lucky me, they couldn't squeeze anything out so they went into several ducts.

This sounds painful beyond belief. But it isn't. Honestly, the ducts seem to open up and allow the cannula to enter relatively pain free. However, my surgeon wanted the cannulas left in place to help guide her to the affected area. So I went down the hall from radiology to surgery with three needles protruding from my left breast. It was quite an experience. I was so thankful my daughter hadn't seen this; it would be an image that would have terrified her to this day.

Only a small incision was needed for the biopsy, nothing a small bandage wouldn't cover. The pain was relative to the size of the cut; meaning it was more of an ache or a burning sensation instead of the unbearable throbbing I'd imagined.

The procedure didn't take long, maybe forty-five minutes, and I was home before noon.

My husband from whom I was separated from at the time, I'll call him Jack, had taken the day off to drive me to and from the hospital. Matt and Robin weren't involved a lot with this procedure; that's the way I wanted it.

When you work in the medical profession, even as a secretary, everyone thinks you have an inordinate amount of medical knowledge. I always felt my family would judge the seriousness of the situation by how I reacted. If I was upset, then it must be bad. So I tried very hard to keep things close, and not show much emotion. Protecting them. I figured that if the biopsy came back okay, I would have eliminated needless anxiety.

Having worked for doctors, I knew that my breast biopsy results would take about five days. So, when day seven came around without any news at all, I was past worry. Waiting is always the hardest part.

I was oblivious to so much of what happened in the early stages. I guess that's a good thing.

The call to my surgeon's office provided no relief. They were at the mercy of the lab where the tissue had been sent.

I waited another day or two then decided to take things into my own hands. Knowing which lab did the pathology for the hospital, I simply called the lab.

No, patients can't normally call the lab and get their results; everything has to go through the doctor. So, I said I was from the doctor's office.

I NEVER said I was from the *surgeon's* office. I plainly stated the name of the doctor I *worked for*. If they misinterpreted the information, so be it. Desperation was setting in, and I was willing to try anything to get some news.

The receptionist was very helpful. "It looks like it's been sent out for further evaluation," she said. "We should have the report soon."

When I asked which local lab it had been sent to, thinking I might call them next, she simply stated "Memorial Sloan Kettering in New York."

My heart skipped a beat, and I took a moment to catch my breath. If the pathologist sent samples of my tissue to Memorial Sloan Kettering, a world famous cancer institute, well, that said it all.

Approximately fourteen days after my biopsy I received the call from my surgeon. Driving down Greenville Avenue in rush hour traffic, my cell phone started ringing. Keeping one eye on the road while the other identified the caller, I hit the talk button.

"You have cancer," she said, confirming what I'd already figured out. "The good news," she quickly added, "is that it's a rare type called cystic hyper-secretory carcinoma, a kind that spreads slowly, and we found it in the very early stages"

In the following minutes she relayed to me that it would need to come out, and she instructed me to contact her office the follow-ing day and schedule a surgery time.

When I hung up the phone my first thought was, "I'm going to throw up." My second thought was, "I have about thirty minutes to figure out how to tell my kids their mom has cancer."

Telling The Kids

Surely, they would notice if I was hiding something. If my face showed any of the emotions, I was trying to control—panic, fear, and failure—it was bound to scare them to death.

I felt that if I told Matt and Robin straight out, showed them I was okay with the idea and I was ready to fight the disease, they would be okay too.

Not everyone takes this approach. And, again, who really knows if there is a correct way to handle it? But I believed they needed to know what I was facing so they would understand if I started freaking out.

Some women choose to keep the diagnosis to themselves for a while; whether it's so they can digest the information before they discuss it, or because they feel it may be too much for their loved ones to handle. Basically, it boils down to doing whatever helps you get through the shock of having cancer and moving onto the next step.

When I arrived home, Robin was the only one there. She was in her room watching television when I went in and sat on the edge of her bed. "I got my pathology results back today," I told her.

She took the remote control and turned the volume down, indicating she was ready to hear what I had to say.

"The doctor told me it's cancer," I said. Then quickly added, "she doesn't think it's bad though."

Robin shrugged her shoulders,

and replied, "Okay," then turned the volume back up. I had been dismissed.

Since I'd never delivered that type of news before, I really hadn't known what to expect. But it wasn't *that*.

I still laugh now when my mom talks about how I reacted. But I know, now, that ignoring it doesn't make it go away.

In my mind, I had pictured a nice mother-daughter talk; one of those heart-to-heart kinds where you say sweet words of encouragement and pledge your undying love to one another. But I figured she had to deal with it in her own way, just as I would, so I let it go.

However, being a mom, I couldn't just let it hang there too long. Surely, Robin was worried or scared and needed consoling. After all, she had just been told her mom had cancer. It was inevitable she'd have questions. So when she walked through the living room later I blurted out, "Robin, I'm not going to die."

She didn't even look at me, just said, "Okay," again, and went back to her room.

Me, I sat in the living room the rest of the evening wondering if I could have handled it better, praying that God would see us through.

I remember just walking out of the room. My first reaction to the news that my mom had cancer was no reaction at all. Looking back though, I think that's the only way I could handle it. I didn't think about it at all, didn't talk about it, and wished half the time that I didn't even know about it.

I should stop here and tell you that I'm hearing some of Robin's thoughts, like the one above, for the first time. We've kept these feelings and fears inside for ten years, which is one of the reasons we're writing this book—to encourage communication. *You can't deal with the unknown. Get it out in the open.*

Next was the task of telling Matt. Admittedly, I was concerned, since I hadn't done well with Robin, but as soon as he got home, I went to his room to get it over with.

"Well," he said, as soon as I told him, "what are you going to do about it?"

"I'm going to fight it. Have it removed and do whatever I need to do," I replied.

He looked up at me and simply stated, "It looks like you have a plan then." That's all he said. That's the kind of person Matt is, though. Black and white. If you have a problem, you address it and take care of business. I knew then he'd be okay.

Making Plans

How could I have told Robin that I wouldn't die? What if I couldn't keep that promise? I mean, I knew God answered prayers. But I also knew dying was just a part of the life cycle. Sometimes good people died, no matter how many prayers had been prayed.

Well, it was time to plan my future, *and* theirs, just in case.

Knowing what I was up against

14

would help me focus. So I started thinking of the worse case scenario. *Death*.

I wasn't real worried when Mom went in for her biopsy, because I was in denial I guess. I just kept thinking, "Oh, she'll be fine, nothing is going to happen." Then, when we found out it was cancer, it was such a shock; I had always been so sure nothing would happen to my mom and that she would never be sick, because I needed her there too bad. And then it started to sink in... the thought of her not being there, and just the possibility that that could happen was so scary.

Being a single mom, raising the kids totally on my own, my foremost concern was their well-being; their fathers hadn't been in the picture for some time and were not a viable option should something happen to me. I called my oldest brother Jonathan and asked if he and his wife, Marcia, would care for the children in my absence. Knowing they loved my kids, and were willing to provide for and support them if I was no longer able, gave me the peace of mind I needed to go forward.

Matt was the man of the family, so it was time to have a serious talk and tell him about the plans I'd made. He didn't want to hear it, but he understood my need to tell him. Patiently he listened as I explained my conversation with his Uncle Jon. Next, I informed him where my financial information could be found. And I finished our talk by assuring him my life insurance would provide for him and Robin, if necessary.

With a sweet hug and a kiss on the top of the head, he told me they'd be okay. So, with the future of my children settled, at least in my mind, I was ready to face any surgery and subsequent therapy necessary to fight the battle.

Mom didn't tell me until years later that she'd had a serious talk with Matt. That would've made it too real to me—her making plans in case she wasn't around anymore.

Matt certainly handled things different than I did!

Contacting my friends and co-workers next, I began gathering opinions on lumpectomy versus mastectomy, names of plastic surgeons, and information on reconstruction techniques.

That left me with only one problem: occupying my mind so I wouldn't give in to self-pity. I couldn't allow my despair and depression to creep in, I had to be strong for my family. As long as I wasn't appearing worried or distraught, they'd be okay. But if they saw even one chink in my armor, they might dwell on what could happen.

I don't think that I ever saw my mom scared. I knew she was concerned, obviously, but she just kept telling me, "I'm gonna be okay." So her acting as if she knew everything was going to be all right caused me not to be so alarmed. At the time, I felt like I had nothing to be worried about...on the surface. I was worried underneath though.

One thing that really helped me

keep my sanity was that I had a friend who was a 'reader.' Brenda loaned me some of her mysteries, and right away, I was hooked. The books allowed me to lose myself in the puzzle between the pages. Many long evenings at home alone, while Matt and Robin were out with their friends, were spent immersed in the lives of amateur sleuths or serial killers; leaving no time for feeling sorry for myself or worrying about the future.

IT'S ABOUT TAKING ACTION

Options

A lumpectomy, or wide-excision biopsy, is when the surgeon makes a cut, removes the area of abnormal cells, and hopefully gets clean margins. Margins are how they refer to the outer edges of the tissue they take. If a microscopic evaluation of the biopsy edges shows normal cells, they know they got all the cancer. If even one area still has cancerous cells showing, they didn't get it all.

Robin woke up at five o'clock in the morning and drove me to the hospital for my lumpectomy; Jack didn't want to miss work for this surgery. If he couldn't make time for me while I was facing a diagnosis of cancer, I knew I would never again have the feelings I once had for him. So, from that point on, I didn't reflect on lost love, I concentrated on ME.

I could've asked my parents to drive me, but I didn't want to worry them. After all, Robin appeared to be handling it okay and didn't seem to mind taking me. Matt, well, I don't know why I didn't ask him. Maybe because he was in high school and I felt he needed to concentrate. Or, maybe it was just that I needed to be with my little girl. I'm not sure.

What makes lumpectomies tricky is that not all abnormal cells are visible to the naked eye. Leaving the surgeon basically cutting blind.

In my case, the tissue all looked the same. My doctor had to guess at how much breast tissue to remove since she couldn't identify where the cancer was. Even so, after the lumpectomy she told me she was ninety-nine percent sure she got it all. Though a large section of tissue was removed, the surgery was still relatively painless. The excision site was covered by 2x2-gauze pad, and extra strength Tylenol relieved the soreness.

However, once I got home, around noon, I started having

aches in my chest muscles, the ones that extended up to my shoulder. This was a sensation I hadn't had with my first surgery, but I thought it was a result of the larger excision made for this procedure.

By early evening, panic took over. While I'd spent all day trying to prove to myself how strong and tough I was, my breast had ballooned up. The pain had spread to my chest wall and I could hardly move my left arm. It was time to call the doctor, and time to call someone to take me to the hospital. Because Robin and Matt were out doing their own thing, I called Jack. He lived nearby, and answered the phone.

By the time I arrived at the emergency room, my breast had tripled its normal size and was showing no signs of stopping the rapid growth. The surgeon informed me I probably had a bleeder and was rushing me straight into the operating room to open up the incision and repair any damage. At that point, my fear had turned from me to my kids. I was worried about reaching them so they'd know where

I was. Luckily, just before I went under, we got Robin on her cell phone, she was at the hospital when I woke up from anesthesia.

Free-flowing blood into my breast had accounted for the swelling and pain. However, the bleeder had been sewn up and I would get to go home the next morning.

The fact that I hadn't been able to reach Robin until late that evening had never crossed my mind again until I started writing this book. I never felt it was her job to sit by my side and care for me. But when I recently asked her if she remembered that evening and what she thought when she found out I'd gone to the hospital, this is what she had to say:

How could I forget? I was at a Rockwall Yellowjacket football game in Mesquite and you were trying to call me. I was there with my best friend, Lisa, watching a player that I liked. I think I saw you calling and didn't pick up the first time because I knew you would want me to leave and I didn't want to. I didn't want to have to tell anyone about you being sick; it's like I was embarrassed. I finally called you back, and you had called Jack to come get you. Isn't that awful? I was so self-ish.

Anyway, I tried not to think about it, and obviously I didn't want to be inconvenienced in any way, because that would mean that something was different or wrong. That and I knew it had to be bad news.

It's important for you to know that I never felt Robin was being selfish. In fact, I didn't realize she felt that way either. In my mind, she was just doing what any kid her age would do. After all, she had a life.

Returning home from getting my bleeder fixed placed me back into another waiting game; wondering if the lumpectomy was successful. My doctor had gone out of town when the pathology report arrived at her office, but I convinced her nurse to fax me a copy of the news.

At twelve noon on October 3,

1995, just as OJ Simpson was receiving his not-guilty verdict, my fax machine started ringing. I didn't spend time reading the entire report, because what I wanted to know was summed up at the bottom under CONCLUSION—three margins still were not clear.

After two surgeries, I still had cancer.

OJ Simpson was free; I had just been given a possible life sentence.

The funny thing, though, Robin was again with me. Right by my side. Literally. She did part-time work in my office and was sitting next to me when the fax came in. And she doesn't even remember that moment.

The options then facing me were to have another lumpectomy: removing even more tissue (after having had two surgeries by then my breast had already become quite misshapen) and having my surgeon again playing a guessing game, possibly still not getting clear margins. Or, I could have a mastectomy: completely removing the cancer and moving on with my life.

My plastic surgeon told me

women deal with breast cancer in one of two ways. Either they will give up, letting their life fill with anger, despair, and self-pity, or they will fight with everything they have.

I chose to fight.

My Choice

Having a mastectomy was an easy choice. Sure, I was a single thirty-five year old woman with hopes of future romance. But that didn't matter. The vanity issue never really bothered me. It was much more important to think about waking up never having to worry if the surgeon had gotten it all.

The next choice was whether I wanted a replacement breast or not. Although many women choose to go sans breast, I knew I wanted something there. Just the thought of getting a replacement made the whole cancer trauma easier for me.

Having my mom lose a breast wasn't ever a big concern of mine because she told me that they were reconstructing it. I was worried about her losing her life! I never

gave a thought to her not having a breast. I didn't think that far ahead.

Several different procedures can be used to reconstruct the breast. Some use implants, a silicone shell filled with either a saline (salt water) solution or a silicone gel. Others use a "flap" of tissue from another part of the body, such as the abdomen or back, either alone or with an implant.

One such flap, *and the option I took*, is called a TRAM flap. TRAM stands for Transverse Rectus Abdominus Muscle, a muscle in the lower abdomen, between the pubic bone and the waist. Tissue (skin, fat and muscle) is taken from the lower abdomen, similar to a "tummy tuck." The tissue is then slid up through a tunnel under the skin to the chest area and formed into a natural-looking breast. A second, minor surgery is needed to reconstruct the nipple and areola. In a *traditional TRAM flap* procedure, the moved tissue remains attached to its original site. The blood vessels are not cut, so the tissue retains its own blood supply.

I would *like* to say that I chose the TRAM flap because abdominal tissue feels most like a natural breast to anyone touching it. But I'll be truthful and admit that vanity MAY have played a small part in my decision. And that's okay. Because if I was going to have to lose my breast, well, by God, I deserved a tummy tuck!

My surgery itinerary was set: go shopping for hospital-wear with my mom on Monday (to show her I was okay and not scared); the mastectomy and reconstruction, an eight to ten hour surgery, would be Tuesday; Wednesday through Saturday would be days spent recuperating in the hospital; and Sunday I would go home and have all the bad stuff behind me (if I got discharged before noon, I would be home in time to see the Dallas Cowboy's game).

A word of wisdom—while going through this process, it's important to have goals. For me, it was planning the surgery right away with the goal of having the surgery behind me quickly, so I would

27

be well healed before Thanksgiving (five weeks after my surgery date.) I wanted to be walking straight, with color back in my cheeks, when the family gathered for Thanksgiving dinner.

These were small goals, but they helped nonetheless. The only flaw in my plan was that I was in the hospital on Matt's eighteenth birthday. I've regretted that decision ever since, and if I had it to do over I'd wait a week.

On the morning of the 'big day' Robin again made the early drive with me, arriving at Presbyterian Hospital of Dallas at five-thirty a.m. My parents met me in the holding area at six-thirty and spent a few minutes encouraging me before I was taken into the operating room. Matt joined them later in the day.

I was tired, a little nervous, but ready to get underway when the attendant wheeled me off. By then an IV had been started and the sedative was beginning to relieve me of the anxiety I had been experiencing, *worrying how long I was going to be under anesthesia*.

How would my family pass the time? Would they be consumed with worry?

Knowing someone else would be controlling my every breath for the next eight to ten hours had also been weighing heavy on my mind. In fact, it was the main thing I'd been afraid of. But my faith, and knowing God would be in control, helped calm my fears, and I was able to go to sleep knowing I was in God's hands, not just the anesthesiologist's.

While I was being opened up like a side of beef, my parents watched the waiting room TV, visited the hospital gift shop, and made several coffee trips to the cafeteria. Matt came and hung out with them for a while, then left, but came back later to see me when I woke up. Robin was restless. She came and went all during the day, going on drives, listening to music, escaping reality.

The day of surgery, I remember being at the hospital for a long time with my grandparents. I remember my Aunt Nancy being there, but I don't remember Matt being there. I know I stayed at the hos-

29

pital for a while, and then drove around a lot, past the mall, to no place in particular.

At some point, I guess someone took me home. Maybe I drove myself home? I honestly don't remember if I was there when my mom woke up or not.

After ten hours, the plastic surgeon met with my family and told them I'd been taken to the recovery room. But...he couldn't feel a pulse in the graft site (where they had created a new breast to replace the one they re-moved). He told them he needed to go back into surgery to see why the blood flow had stopped; which meant I'd be spending a couple more hours under the knife.

"I knew you had to go back in," Robin told me. *"But whoever was telling me that stuff made it sound like everything was going to be okay. I never thought you WOULDN'T be okay—just because I couldn't have handled thinking that."*

Actually, I remember waking up

in recovery for a few minutes with the plastic surgeon telling me we were going back in. It didn't matter though; I was in no condition to go anywhere else.

When I woke up three hours later, I was being wheeled to my room with my family around me. The only thing I remember saying was. "I feel thinner already."

One Day at a Time

Hospital stays are never pleasant, so I won't dwell on those five days. As expected, I felt bad, took pain pills, slept when I could, and walked when they made me.

My family was wonderful because they understood I really wanted to be left alone; we picked one day (Friday) when I thought I'd be up to seeing guests and they all visited at that time.

It was also that very Friday night that I remember crying in front of someone for the first time during the whole ordeal. Around eight o'clock, after everyone had gone home, my general surgeon, Dr. Elizabeth Naftalis, came to my room while making rounds. She said, "I stopped by my office before coming up here, and I'm glad I did because *this* was waiting for me." She nodded toward the document in front of her; she was holding my future in her hands.

"We got it all," she assured me.

Dr. Naftalis then walked to my bed and hugged me as I cried.

Once she left, I tried to compose myself before making any phone calls. You see, even then I was trying to be stoic. Be the brave, fearless one. I called my mom and gave her the news. So much for stoic—we *both* cried!

In retrospect, I think I called my mom first because I needed more time to gather my composure. Telling my children I would live to torment them for years to come was going to be emotional for me; I'd been waiting four weeks to be able to say those words to them, and the moment had finally come.

Now it would make for a much better story if I could tell you something really awesome took place. However, the moment went by

relatively uneventful. Robin answered the phone, and when I tried
to get the words out all I could
do was get choked up. Which worried her, because she hadn't heard
or seen me cry about it. When I
finally said, "They got it all"
she offered a few words of encouragement. Things like, "That's
good," and "You'll be okay." But I
never asked her what she felt when
I told her. So I asked her now.

*I vaguely remember you calling
and telling me. I think during
that time, and for some years after, I never wanted to talk about
it or think about it, so now I
don't have a lot of specific memories about the calls or instances.*

When I told Matt, he took it in
stride. Why wouldn't he? He'd
known all along that it would be
okay.

My mom and dad came up the
night before my discharge from the
hospital to pick up many of the
flowers I'd received and take them
to my apartment. I'd received a
LOT.

It was funny because when I first thought about the hospital I was afraid that I wouldn't have any flowers; I had always kept to myself and had only a small circle of friends. However, I was very surprised. I received cards and flowers from people I hadn't spoken to in years. So many flowers, in fact, that my room was overflowing and I began having the nurses share some with other patients who weren't so lucky.

Thinking of this still brings a smile to my face. Knowing that so many people cared is a special feeling. And it wasn't the gifts themselves; it was truly the *thoughts* that counted.

In addition to clearing the room of plants, I spent the night before my discharge learning how to take care of the bandages across my breast and the ones stretched across my abdomen. My nurse also took extra time to teach me how to care for the three drains that were left in my breast and stomach; they would be going home with me.

Just a quick note about drains. When a space is created in the body where there used to be tissue, your body's natural response is to fill the space with fluid. The soft tube-like drains, placed during surgery, have a bulb at the end to collect the excess fluid. When the amount of drainage decreases to a point where the body can absorb the fluid, the drains are removed. Until then, you have to measure the fluid that's collected in the bulb and keep the surgical incisions clean and protected.

I went home with three drains in place: one in my breast just under the incision; one in my pubic area, under the abdominal incision; and one close to my navel, above the abdominal incision.

The drains! I remember seeing them on my mom and watching her clean them. They didn't bother me that bad; I think because I knew that she was taking care of them, and I didn't have to touch them. In fact, I don't ever remember Mom asking me to help with them—which I still feel so bad about now, that she had to do all of that herself and had no one there to help. She was all by herself, in pain, and managing everything on her own, just like she always had. Thinking about this still makes me cry. But I know she did everything for herself because she didn't want me and Matt to feel burdened in any way. She wanted us to keep going along like normal kids.

Robin was, again, the designated driver. She sat with me as I very impatiently waited to be released. She even took my prescription for painkillers to the pharmacy down the street and had it filled so we'd be able to go straight home as soon as the nurses let me leave.

This was when you got mad at me for not getting the car inspected; when you got in the car and saw the sticker hadn't been changed. The ONE thing you asked me to do, and I just ended up blowing the money. You got over it right away; I guess you realized I was too preoccupied.

Once home, Robin made sure I

was carefully positioned on the sofa, ready for the Cowboy's game. Then she brought a fresh glass of ice water and set it down on the end table beside my bottle of medicine. She confirmed that I could walk to the bathroom by myself and tend the drains.

Because it was important for me to show everyone how tough I was, I was determined to be back at work four weeks after surgery, instead of the customary six. To reach that goal, I spent the first week at home resting and the next two getting up and walking around the apartment. Walking straighter and more upright each day.

Cancer was now behind us, the only tale-tell sign was potted plants on all the end tables and gauze pads on the bathroom shelf.

And, finally, the day came when I was able to return to work; yes, right at four weeks post-op as planned. It was a day I actually enjoyed very much. All my co-workers gathering round to give me their congratulations and welcome me back. What was funny, though, was watching as they all tried to catch a peek at my breast, seeing if they could tell which one was real. I didn't blame them though, I knew I was a novelty; at least for a day.

Before long the drains came out, the pain was gone, and I no longer looked like I had gone through a life-changing ordeal. People took for granted that strength I had so badly wanted to show them. I was well and everything was normal. For the time being.

What I didn't know then was that I would think about having cancer every day for the rest of my life; that no matter how 'well' I looked, cancer, and my health, always haunted me; and that each day that passed would bring new doubts and fears to Robin.

IT'S ABOUT WARNING SIGNS

Anxiety

As Robin said earlier, talking about my cancer wasn't an option for her. It was the very last thing she wanted to do. Even though the news was good and they had gotten it all, it wasn't mentioned.

We didn't even talk about how blessed we were that the mastectomy had gotten all the cancer, and gotten it early. It hadn't spread. Which meant that I didn't have to have radiation or chemotherapy. I realized how incredibly lucky I was, but, again, Robin didn't mention it—I didn't know if she was even aware that I had gotten off very easy!

Almost imperceptibly, she began withdrawing, cutting off all communication with her family and her friends. She just wanted to be in her room, where no one could bother her or ask if she was okay. Was this normal adolescent behavior or warning signs of something much deeper?

Soon the very thought of having to leave the comfort and security of the apartment, and more specifically her bedroom, brought on severe panic attacks. And before long, depression and anxiety kept her stomach in knots, causing her to throw up every time she attempted to eat (her 5'3" frame rapidly dropping to skin and bones.) She was even unable to seek solace from sleep, as the still of the night only magnified her fear of losing me.

What could I do to help her when I didn't even know what was going on? How could I get counseling or treatment for her if I couldn't get her out of the house? Had I spent over a year and multiple surgeries trying to hang on to my life, only to end up losing my daughter?

I'm not sure of the date, but it was during my sophomore year when I really withdrew. It was just a few weeks, I think, after I found out about my mom's cancer.

I would get very emotional and overwhelmed by EVERYTHING, and start crying at the drop of a hat.

My nerves had been on edge earlier in the year, probably hormones and high school. But my mom's cancer pushed me over the edge.

Then, the more emotionally upset I became, the more I felt like people were looking at me. Wondering what was wrong with me. I just wanted so bad to be able to be normal and not have such heavy things on my mind. I wanted to be superficial like everyone else.

For a while I attended the laid-back classes, like photojournalism and technical theater. But one day I had a started getting emotional in photojournalism, and had to run to the bathroom to cry. When I never showed back up, the teacher sent someone in to check one me. I was so humiliated. Instead of returning to class, I went to the nurse's office and stayed there until class was over.

That was when I started skipping school, because I didn't want to be put on the spot by anyone. I *didn't want to be in class, or have to explain to the teacher why I needed to leave if I got upset.*

Not until the nurse at the high school called me, did I realize Robin was becoming so emotional.

It's hard to see emotion when someone won't talk to you about anything.

But I explained to the nurse about the cancer and hoped she would be able to help assuage Robin's fear if it happened again.

By the end of my sophomore year, the panic attacks and the fear of having the attacks, became debilitating. Which caused me to stop going to school altogether—and basically stay in my room all the time.

When I could no longer get Robin to go to school, I called the school counselor and asked for guidance. We discussed the possibility of school sponsored home-schooling for Robin to get her education requirements in.

Remember, this was back in the 1990's, the trend of everyone home-schooling their children wasn't as easy as it is now.

Also, keep in mind I was trying to be very careful about forcing her into doing something to further upset her emotional state.

However, the school counselor told me that unless Robin had a medical condition, or unless she had a psychologist's note stating she was mentally impaired, home school wasn't an option.

Again, Robin wouldn't talk to anyone about how she was feeling or what she was going through. And she was adamant against going to a doctor or therapist. Honestly, at that point, I didn't realize how serious her panic attacks had become. Not that it mattered, I doubt I could have done anything, anyway. But the point is—I didn't have an official medical excuse for her behavior to show the school.

Suffice to say that after several discussions with the high school, pleading for their consideration and assistance, it only resulted in them filing truancy charges on me and Robin. She then forced to go before a judge to explain why she wouldn't go to school, and I was being held responsible for, basically, being irresponsible.

The local judge, however, showed compassion. After hearing our story, and that we had sought support and alternatives from the school (the counselor confirmed we had,) he directed us to a privately sponsored homeschool program to get Robin through graduation.

We got the books. Began an at-home curriculum. And I thought we had overcome a hurdle. I mistakenly thought I had made things easier for my troubled little girl.

Isolation

Matt was in his final year of high school. He had a life, and I rarely saw him.

Robin was staying busy. Working part-time at the medical office I managed, and working on her home schooling at night.

She would go to her room as soon as we got home from work, and she would stay there most of the

44

night.

I spent a lot of time alone in my room. It kept me from having to talk to anyone, face anything. It's kind of embarrassing, but when I was alone in my room, with my stereo turned up, I would sing along and try to pretend I was somewhere else.

Without the kids around, I got real lonesome and decided it would be nice to have someone to do things with. So I started talking to a single neighbor, we struck up a friendship, and we became an item.

Matt didn't seem to mind, and Robin acted indifferent. At least until Jeff and I became serious!

When I told Robin that Jeff and his sixteen-year-old daughter, Molly, would be moving in with us, she got upset. She didn't want them there. She used all kinds of excuses for trying to get me to change my mind and not let them come.

Knowing I was making a decision that could possibly upset her delicate balance even more than it already was difficult. I love Robin and Matt above everything else, but I had to determine where to draw the line on my own happiness.

The discussion was settled—Jeff and Molly would be joining our family; with a promise to Robin that she was more important to me than anything, and if things became unbearable, if everyone wasn't getting along after a few months time, we would decide what needed to be done to keep our family happy.

I had pretty much stopped all contact with my friends by the time Jeff and Molly moved in. That was a real bad time for me. Not just because of them. I was upset all the time anyway. But when they moved in wasn't too long after we found out my mom was going to be all right, and I really needed her then.

I didn't want to talk to her about things, but I wanted her to be there just for ME whenever I needed her. The thought that someone else might be getting her time and attention made me mad.

Some nights I remember wishing she would come in and comfort me while I was crying, so we could talk about things and she would know how I was feeling. But I never would let her, anyway. I would tell her I was okay and didn't want to be bothered.

Jeff and I used to call Robin my "stealth" daughter. She would move around the house without being seen, leaving only a shadow in her path, or a wisp of a sound behind her.

But the panic attacks she had experienced in school appeared to have subsided since homeschooling began, so we thought she just wanted her space. Neither of us had any idea she was upstairs, just above us, scared and in tears.

Alarm

It took about six months from the time Jeff and I got married, until Robin's symptoms became evident to us. She stopped going to work, had completely cut off all communication with her best friend, and was dropping weight daily (or so it appeared).

Even though I wanted to be with my mom, I still couldn't bear going to work with her and having to face anyone with their questions about school, how I was feeling, and so on. Although, I missed her terribly.

I remember that I often watched out the window as she left for work, crying as she drove away. For some reason I worried a lot about her getting in an accident. Maybe it was just that I didn't want to think that anything else would happen to her, and as long as she was home she was safe.

But, for whatever reason, I would always think of Mom going to work and not coming back. And I would pray so hard that she would be safe.

It sounds weird now, even to me, but I never worried when she had to go back to the surgeon for follow-ups. Maybe because she never made a big deal of it, and because I think that in the back of my mind I knew the doctors would always take care of her. But I think I worried about a car wreck so much because then there wouldn't be anyone there for her.

When she went to the doctor it was controlled, and I knew she would be okay. But if she were in some freak accident, well, that was out of everyone's control.

Yes, somehow everything always comes back to control. Even now, in fact... But back then I especially needed to control who I saw and where I went. And I guess I felt scared and helpless if I couldn't control what happened to my mom.

The only time Robin would leave her room would be when no one was home. Then she might even venture out and go driving around, listening to the radio. But never with anyone.

Her anxiety had gotten her to the point that she could no longer hide the symptoms from me. She could no longer eat without vomiting, because her stomach was in knots with worry. She couldn't sleep at night because of her fear. And she was no longer able to keep the crying from me; it had gotten so she couldn't control it.

The hardest part of going through the fear and anxiety was that I just didn't know why I was sad all the time. My mom was cancer free, nothing was wrong with her anymore. So why was I still so upset?

It was a particularly difficult time for me because I felt desperate. I wanted to stay home and comfort her, but I had just gotten a new job and had to be there. Not to mention that it was a financial low point, and we needed every penny we could get.

But I took advantage of working around doctors and I went to the psychologist at the hospital where I worked and told her about my daughter. Her response was, "This is a very serious situation. You need to get her to see someone immediately, and she probably needs to be hospitalized."

I didn't know that!

I never told this to Robin before, because it wouldn't have helped the situation any. It was something I just had to pray about...

However, because I had just started a new job, I was in-between insurance benefits. So, not only did I feel like a failure for letting the situation get so out of control, but I didn't have the money to get medical help for my daughter.

For weeks we struggled through as best we could. Robin stayed at home by herself most of the time. Some days, though, she would take me to work so she could keep the car. Having that small bit of control helped her.

She would even watch daytime television looking for answers. Searching for someone who was going through what she was.

Believe it or not, Oprah did have a guest speaker, a physician, who specialized in social anxiety. Robin told me about him (she'd taken notes because she felt like he was describing her), so I tried to contact him. He charged an astronomical fee for counseling, so that was a dead-end, but Robin had kept the name of his book and asked me to buy it for her. She even read it. And while it did address some of the fear she was having, it was like putting a band aide on an amputation.

At night, when her desperation was more than she could bear, she would wake me up and I would go to her room and sit with her. This had become a several-nights-a-week occurrence. Sometimes I'd stroke her hair and try to get her to sleep. But mostly I'd just reassure her that I was okay. And, of course, I prayed. A lot!

The anxiety and all the fear always came on worse at night. I think it was just the fact of not having anyone around and having no distractions. I couldn't really make myself think of anything else except my distress.

A lot of times at night, when it was late, I would leave my television on a channel that just played instrumental music; it would also have scriptures on and off, with pictures of lakes and trees in the background. Some nights that would help me go to sleep.

But one night I remember waking

my mom up and asking her how we knew that our faith in God, and the way we believed, was right.

She told me that she believed because 'she needed to.' She couldn't make it through the day without the promise of God watching over us, helping us. She needed to pray, talk to God, and share her innermost thoughts and fears with Him. And if she was wrong, and there wasn't really a God, well, the belief of one had given her a lifetime of comfort and hope.

I told her my fear of losing her, and also of my grandparents dying. It sounds silly now. But Mom reminded me that the natural progression would be for them to die before us. And, while we would miss them, they would have lived their lives for God and weren't afraid of dying. It would be their final accomplishment, going to Heaven, seeing Jesus, and then meeting up with all their loved ones who had gone before them.

Being reminded of this somehow helped. Knowing Nanaw, my great-grandmother, would be waiting for them gave me a sense of peace.

I think those nights were a real important time for me; getting closer to God, praying all the time, and trying to have faith that He would keep my mom safe and that He would help me get better.

IT'S ABOUT TAKING BACK YOUR LIFE

Face your fears

I truly believe that once Robin started talking about her fears, she started getting better emotionally and physically. No, it wasn't overnight, but it was baby steps.

Oftentimes, when I left for work, she'd want me to drop her off to spend the day at her grandparents. Her heart-to-heart talks with her grandparents (Nanny and Pappaw) helped her a lot.

You see, my parents have always offered unconditional love. They never make judgments. So, it was, and still is, always very easy to go to them and talk about anything in the world.

Robin could talk to Nanny, or not talk at all and just watch TV with her. Or sometimes Nanny and Pappaw would pray with Robin, which help calmed her a lot. They would share their faith, study the Bible, and show Robin exactly why they weren't afraid of dying, or of anything.

I would call my grandparents in the middle of the night or early in the morning—just so they could pray with me.

Again, this process took time. But as long as you see some progress, you hold on to that hope.

Another thing that I believed helped a lot, but that Robin doesn't actually remember too much about now, was St. John's Wort.

Let me put in this disclosure, so to speak, about how you should definitely seek medical attention any time you have medical problems. But, even though things were better, I couldn't get Robin to agree to see a doctor. She was fighting so hard to be normal that even suggesting a counselor, psychologist, or medical doctor would shake the foundation she was rebuilding. So we went unconventional for a while.

Jeff's daughter, Molly, was working at GNC during this time.

GNC-General Nutrition Centers— is a retail chain of health products. One October evening she came in with a huge book about vitamin supplements. At the time I thought it was coincidental, but now I believe Molly brought it in because she thought it might offer help; which it did!

Having worked in the medical field for most of my adult life, I just knew that if I could find something to help ease some of the anxiety Robin was feeling, she could begin healing. And once her level of anxiety was diminished, maybe she would agree to see a doctor.

So, with Molly's book in hand, I searched through the index for depression. Then I cross-referenced the depression herbs with ones that were indexed under stomach ailments also. And this is what I found.

St John's Wort's therapeutic effects are found to include:

- *Relieves mild to moderate anxiety and depression.*
- *Promotes restful sleep.*

- *Improves capillary circulation.*
- *Increases cardiac circulation.*
- *Eases gastrointestinal distress.*
- *Relieves discomfort associated with premenstrual syndrome.*
- *Fights retroviruses.*

Three of those were right on target, so the next time Molly went to work, she came home with a bottle of St. John's Wort for Robin.

I don't remember St. John's Wort helping as much as my mom remembers it did. But maybe I just couldn't see it like she could.

While Robin doesn't remember it, Jeff and I will always swear that it was a catalyst to the road to recovery. Within a couple weeks after taking it, Robin was wasn't as emotional. She even stopped throwing up as much. I considered it our answer to prayer.

The Christmas before I turned seventeen, I remember I was feeling a little better, and I started talking on the phone to my best friend, Lisa, again. I had gone a long time without talking to her.

I also started going a few places with her. But I didn't really start getting a lot better until I started dating Mike.

I remember Robin being so much better at this point. Maybe she wasn't, and I thought she was, or maybe she just doesn't remember. But, she was acting almost like her old, happy self. She was still feeling the anxiety, but was able to somewhat control it.

Again, back to the control issue. As long as Robin could control who she talked to, where she went, and that she was always the driver, her anxiety was relatively low.

Things were moving quickly, Robin was gaining courage. And Lisa even introduced Robin to a 'guy.'

I can't remember how they knew him, or anything. Just that I was very worried, because I knew Robin wouldn't tell anyone about the anxiety she still felt, so I was afraid going out with a stranger might push her back into depression.

In fact, Robin never really

told Lisa everything that was going on with her.

Plus, to top everything off, my son and his best friend told me the guy Robin was interested in hung out with people who were 'no good.'

Well, I expected Matt to rag on anyone Robin would be interested in. But when Mike, Matt's best friend for over seven years at that point, agreed, well I took it seriously. Mike never said too much, and what he said wasn't usually judgmental.

It especially worried me when Mike mentioned it again the next time he came to see Matt. So I told Mike if he was really concerned about Robin, maybe HE should ask her out.

Well, I'll spare you some of the details, but after a little more of my prying, and after Mike asked Matt if he could date his sister, Mike and Robin were set up to go out on their first date.

I didn't think it would be too bad. They'd known each other for years. But back came the anxiety.

You should know that Mike had no clue what Robin had gone

through, because, basically, Matt didn't understand everything either, so he never mentioned it to Mike. But we're talking Matt was about nineteen or twenty at this point, so if his little sister was weepy, depressed, or getting sick to her stomach all the time, it was too much information.

When Mike came to pick up Robin, she was in her room vomiting, crying, and wanting to back out.

Since Mike was in the living room waiting, I stepped in and claimed a little of my 'mom control.' I gave him an abbreviated version about her anxiety; only that she had a nervous stomach and got embarrassed about it. He went back to her room and talked to her. A little later that evening they went to his house and watched a Dallas Stars' game. He had wanted to take her to the game but going out was too stressful. She had declined that offer and settled for TV. She needed baby steps. The fear of the impending panic and anxiety was enough to keep her from doing new things.

I didn't really start getting a lot better until Mike and I started going out. There was one night in particular that he was going to baby-sit my second cousin Macy with me. I didn't want him to go, but he wanted to be with me. On the way I had to ask him to pull over because I thought I was going to throw up. I told him, then, about everything, and how I was sick all the time. After I told him, I felt so much better and he really, really helped me.

Then, since I was dating some-one, my mom encouraged me to see a gynecologist. I'd never seen one before and Mom said that by the time you turned eighteen you should have a thorough exam. Plus, she said I needed to have a doctor I was comfortable with in case I decided I wanted birth control; especially since it looked like I was developing a relationship with Mike. I didn't mind talking to my mom about this, we had always talked openly about girl stuff.

Even though Robin was much bet-ter, she still had emotional prob-lems. And she still wouldn't agree to see a psychologist or psychiatrist. So when she started getting fairly serious with Mike, I used that as an opportunity to suggest a gynecologist, knowing one could help her, or at least diagnose how serious her problem might be.

Robin wanted me to be there for her first visit, and I was glad to be. We both went in and explained our visit was two-fold. The doctor listened as Robin and I each told her parts of the story.

Robin had found someone she could talk to. Another answer to prayer.

Going to the doctor made all the difference. Actually, at first my mom did all the talking, I cried a little. But then the doctor shared with me about how her dad had been real sick when she was young. She would wait on the front porch everyday for him to come home. If he was late, she would panic. This helped me relate to her.

It was then that I was diagnosed with depression and put on 50 mg of Zoloft daily.

Sure, I still struggled some

after that, but that was the turning point for me. But the fact that there was a diagnosis and medicine that could help made me feel much better.

What's normal and what isn't

No two people will react the same when they are coping with a serious illness. But, surely, there are correct ways and responses to manage. Robin and I didn't have a clue; maybe there isn't a clue! But if there is, we want to share it so others won't suffer like Robin did.

Hopefully by reading our story, you can already see where we could have improved. Or, you may even be able to identify with some of the symptoms Robin had.

Face it, her reaction—while some consider it normal—was not healthy.

So I went to the experts for the definition of what's normal, what's not, and what are the warning signs.

After all, it's tough enough for someone you love to battle cancer; it shouldn't have the power to claim you, too!

Remember...It's normal to feel angry, sad, scared, lonely, and even guilty, if you are watching and caring for someone who has a serious illness.

But the tricky part is how to tell these normal feelings apart from stress or depression.

Here's some information on warning signs that Robin and I compiled by reviewing a multitude of articles, books, and newsletters. If you find that you relate to, or experience some of these signs, you may want to seek professional guidance. Don't be afraid. It doesn't mean you are crazy or abnormal at all. It just means you have a lot to deal with and may need someone to talk things over with; someone who is impartial and out of the loop.

Warning Signs of Extreme Stress

- Anxiety (nervous, apprehensive)
- Cranky (touchy, irritable)
- Excessive fatigue (feeling bone tired)
- Withdrawn from friends & family
- Sleep problems (sleeping too

much or not enough)
- Increased illnesses (receptive to all colds, bugs, etc. that are going around)
- Unwarranted anger towards the person you care for, your family or yourself

Warning Signs of Depression

- No interest or pleasure in things you usually enjoy
- Sad or unfeeling
- Crying easily or for no reason
- Feeling insignificant, useless, or guilty
- Change in appetite; sudden change in weight
- Trouble concentrating or making decisions
- Memory problems
- Headaches, backaches or digestive problems
- Thoughts of death or suicide

If you have thoughts about death or suicide, please talk to a doctor, a counselor, or your clergy. Don't try to work through your problems by yourself.

IT'S ABOUT LIFE AFTER CANCER

Letting go of guilt

Even though her depression and anxiety were diagnosed and were being treated, she still had trouble managing the source of the problem. Her guilt.

A lot of the crippling anxiety Robin felt, and still feels, is due to guilt over things she believes she should have done differently.

It's tough to let go of the guilt. But until you do, you won't ever be able to move on.

I still cry when I think about not being there for my mom. I know she was sad, physically hurting, and I probably would have been a real comfort to her and kept her company. I still feel very upset about it. I'm learning to not dwell on that, though.

I feel so ashamed of that now, and embarrassed, but I know that my mom has forgiven me. She knew that I never would have made it through any other way. There was no other way for me to cope with it

My mom was so worried about me, and she knew I was better not being there. That's how selfless and generous she is.

Guilt is a terrible thing. But the truth is, all those things Robin feels guilty about—I never gave them a second thought. In fact, I feel guilty for asking her to be so responsible at such a young age.

I honestly feel Robin lost her teenage years because I was sick. She was never allowed to be a crazy adolescent because she had to take care of her mom. Get up at four-thirty in the morning to take me to surgery, sit there by herself while I was under then knife, take me home and put me to bed, and go to the pharmacy to get my medicine and dressings.

Because I was a single mom, she was forced into being my care-

giver. Even though I wasn't inca-
pacitated, I required her to be
there for ME, to take me places,
run errands for me, and to basically give up those happy carefree
adolescent years she should have
been able to enjoy. That was so
unfair of me to do to her.

*I don't think it was unfair of
my mom, and I have never blamed
her for it. It was just the hand
that was dealt to us and shaped
who we are today.*

I still carry a lot of guilt. I
take the blame for the anxiety and
depression she fell into.
However, here is what some of
the professionals say about guilt:
"Feeling guilty is a common reaction for caregivers. You may
worry that you aren't helping
enough, or that your work or dis-
tance from your loved one is getting in the way. You may even feel
guilty that you are healthy. Or
you may feel guilty for not acting
upbeat or cheerful. But know that
it's okay. You have reasons to
feel upset and hiding them may
keep other people from understand-

ing your needs." Taken from **When Someone You Love Is Being Treated for Cancer** by the National Institutes of Health - National Cancer Institute.

The following pages are an excerpt from **Re-labelling Guilt;** an article by Alison McWalter, in the *Alberta Caregivers Association—Bi-Weekly eNews,* No. 17, November 27th, 2004.

What Causes Guilt?

Guilt is a feeling that we all experience at some time. We feel guilty if we think we have not lived up to the standards we set for ourselves, or if we think we have done something wrong. We tell ourselves we 'should' have behaved differently, or that we 'ought' to have done better. Sometimes we may even tell ourselves that we must be a bad person for feeling or acting in this way.

Caregivers may find themselves feeling guilty for all sorts of reasons, depending on their situation and where they are in their caregiving journey. I've given a few examples here, but I know that there are many more.

- Caregivers can experience many difficult feelings as they face the challenges ahead. They may feel tired, overwhelmed, sad, angry, frustrated, trapped, and stressed. Caregivers may then tell themselves that they shouldn't have such feelings, and that this makes them a bad caregiver.

- Caregivers can feel under stress at times, which can lead to them feeling more irritable, snappy, and angry than usual. They may speak more sharply to others, or withdraw from others. Again, they may tell themselves they shouldn't act this way, and feel guilty for doing so.

The Guilt Cycle

When we feel guilty, we can get into a guilt cycle:

- Feeling guilty
- I shouldn't have done this

71

- I'm a bad caregiver
- I shouldn't feel this way

We feel guilty, we tell ourselves we shouldn't act or feel like this, which makes us feel more guilty and so on.

This guilt cycle can drain our energy; it can make us feel almost paralyzed and unable to cope.

Breaking the Guilt Cycle-Re-labelling Guilt

- Recognize your feelings—this is an important first step in dealing with difficult feelings. Since caregivers spend a lot of time looking after others, they often don't pay attention to their own feelings. If we do look at our own feelings, we can look at what is causing us to feel guilty, and try to break the guilt cycle.
- Accept yourself—as a human being you are not perfect; you can and do make mistakes. Accepting that this is part of being human can help you find ways to learn from any mistakes, and move forward. Re-

member, too, that you have many strengths, and give your-self credit for these.

- Re-label the guilt; guilt is paralyzing, it stops us moving forward.
- Watch out for the 'Shoulds'- when you find your-self saying or thinking 'I should have done...,' or 'I shouldn't have done...,' take a moment to stop and reflect. Ask yourself, 'Who says I should?'-are you being too critical of yourself, what would you say to a friend in a similar situation? Sometimes it helps to replace 'should' with 'it would be nice if', for example, instead of saying 'I should always be there to look after my father', you could say ' It would be nice if I could be there to look after my father, what are the ways that I can help?'
- Accept help — remember that as a caregiver, you do not have to do everything. Accepting help does not mean that you are not doing your job; it is okay to share the care.
- Talk to someone—sharing feelings with others (whether

friends, relatives, other caregivers, minister or priest, doctor, counselor) can help you to put these feelings in perspective, or find ways of coping with them.

These are some suggestions to help break the guilt cycle and re-label guilt. Remember that no-one's situation is exactly the same as another's, so it is important to find what works for you. Remember also that as a caregiver, you are important—look after yourself too!

(special thanks to Alison McWalter for allowing us to reprint the above article)

It's okay to move on

There comes a point when you let go of the guilt and let yourself enjoy life. It's okay. You deserve it!

Even with the medicine, it was still a struggle for a while. I took a job at the hospital where my mom worked, a position that re-

quired me to deal with people! And, actually, every day that went by gave me more confidence. Within a few months I had even been promoted to a position in the president's office.

My new position was quite challenging, though, because I had to meet and greet the hospital board members, arrange parties, attend functions. But I know God gave me the strength I needed, because the only time I ever had anxiety was when I had to ride to an event with someone. I felt better driving so I could leave a situation if I was uncomfortable. Usually I could drive myself, even though it may have appeared odd to some people.

During this time my relationship with my mom got back to normal, and I could talk to her about anything and everything.

One of Robin's biggest accomplishments was when she took the job at the hospital. I didn't know how in the world she'd be able to work the front desk for our business office, but she did great.

Then, when she asked to be promoted to a job in administration, I was so proud. She was finding herself.

She thrived in that environment. Although, truth be known, to this day I doubt most people realized what a step of faith and courage it was for her to be there.

After a couple years, however, I believe Robin started feeling some of the stress and pressure that working in an office with other women can often produce. And, since the last thing Robin wanted was to have conflict, she made the decision to move on.

For months, Mike and his mom had talked to me about changing jobs; going to work for her title company. It would mean another promotion. It would reduce my drive to work to only five minutes, which would be cool.

Change was tough though. The thought of leaving what had become familiar to me was scary. I had overcome my fears to get where I was at that job—and I was about to start all over. However, the part that made me the most anxious was having to give my notice to my supervisor.

But, the night before I gave my notice, Mike left a note in my car to be strong. It helped me a lot. I still have that note.

Robin was happy. She had a great new career, a fiancé who treated her like a princess, and more confidence and strength than I could ever remember her having.

From that point, she continued to grow. The only set back, a slight one, was when she and Mike got married. Her nerves got the best of her. I think the week before they got married, she spent a lot of time in tears.

She wasn't afraid to get married. She was afraid to leave the comfort of home; afraid to leave me. Who's not to say this was just normal premarital jitters though?

Me and my mom went to bridal shops, I tried on dresses, and picked out accessories. But I knew there was NO WAY I could go through the anxiety of a big wedding. So Mike and I just eloped to Las Vegas. It was perfect for us;

neither of us like to be the center of attention, so low-key was good.

It's been a long road. But Robin has finally recovered nicely from our breast cancer experience. Robin and Mike have a normal, happy life in the country. She's gotten her escrow license, so her career HAS moved forward. The only fear she experiences now is whether or not she wants kids...she already worries about what she'd do if they came home late!

My life has gotten much better. I think I'm back to what I'd call "normal." Mike and I are married, we built a beautiful house, and we have two sweet puppies. It's still a struggle sometimes. But, hey, LIFE can be a struggle. And whenever I find myself getting emotional, I talk to my mom.

For a long time I continued to try to avoid situations I thought might make me vulnerable to anxiety; like social functions, those kind of things. But I've recently started to face those things head on.

Last year I finally started seeing a psychologist. Being away from my mom and adjusting to marriage was stressing me out. I DID NOT want to go backward and end up where I was. So I reached out and found someone I could open up to.

The psychologist gave me some clarity on the pressure I was putting on myself and made me realize that I realistically couldn't do everything. I always try to do everything myself so it will be done the way I want it done. I guess it goes back to that control issue.

The main thing about the therapist, though, is she was there as someone who was not family and was totally removed from the situation. I could tell her things and then leave her office and not worry about someone's feelings being hurt because everything was in confidence.

She gave me some good ideas, and some things that I wasn't totally on board with. But overall, the experience of therapy helped.

IT'S ABOUT BELIEVING

Sharing Our Faith

When I finished writing the first draft of this book, it didn't feel right. Something was missing. I'd left out a HUGE part of the story—how we were able to make it through with our health and our sense of humor.

You see, I've never been one to talk about my faith. It's something very personal to me, and I guard it very carefully. So when I tell people about my breast cancer, I acknowledge that I had a miracle, but I leave it at that.

Not this time, though!

IT'S ABOUT BELIEVING was added and now I feel we're giving you the entire story.

I believe in God and that he sent Jesus to offer us hope. It's that belief that gives me strength when I'm down, gives me courage when I'm afraid, and makes up a large part of the person I am.

I still pray every night when I go to bed, or when I feel afraid. I believe in angels. And I KNOW someone is always watching over me.

For non-believers this probably sounds pretty hokey. But that's okay. This belief gives me a tremendous peace of mind and helps me face anything I come up against.

Was I scared when I found out I had cancer? YES. But I always felt God was with me and would help me and my family deal with whatever the prognosis would be.

It took three months from the time I first realized I had something wrong, until the day the surgeon said "We got it all." And most of that time I had doubts over whether I would be a survivor. Cancer is random. Who knows why someone gets it, and how bad it will be? But I can honestly tell you that I knew, without any doubt, that God loved me and would help me face breast cancer and everything it entailed with strength and dignity. And no matter what outcome I had, God would be with me and my family, healing our heart and comforting our souls.

I stayed busy, never dwelled or concentrated on the bad things. Although I did find out about every possible thing I might have to face...which wasn't always pretty. But I wanted to know all my options and plan ahead.

The only regret I have is that I didn't go into counseling when I was given my cancer diagnosis. I felt very strongly that our faith and strong family would be all we needed; I did NOT need to talk about my feelings with a bunch of strangers who probably didn't even believe in healing. But I was WRONG.

Asking for help, and learning through the experience of others is not a weakness. You see, God gives counselors, doctors, and nurses a special gift. We need to reach out to them sometimes. We need to admit we're not invincible and use the tools God has supplied us with.

I don't know how I would have gotten through this ordeal without believing in God and knowing that

He is always there. I prayed every night that God would give me peace of mind. The nights when I was up all night crying, I prayed for comfort and that I would be able to let go of the worry and put everything in God's hands and let myself rest. I still pray at night, and as I'm saying my prayers, I always end up drifting off to sleep because of the peace I feel.

I know He wants to bear our burdens so we don't have to. I just really tried to believe that, and every time I would start to feel depressed, I'd say a prayer and turn it over to God. Even to this day I do this. Sometimes troubling thoughts still creep in, like 'what if my mom doesn't come home today' or 'what if something happens to my husband,' but I immediately dismiss them, don't dwell on them, and say a prayer that the people I love are protected, and go on.

Seeing Us Through

I don't know why I survived breast cancer, when there are so many women dying from it. I don't

83

believe God loved me more, or that I had a stronger faith. Again, it's random. A part of God's plan, I guess, even though that feels odd when I say it.

What I DO know is that I have to share what cancer did to us. How it affected our lives. It's a responsibility Robin and I have, to try and help others through our experience.

The journey has definitely made us stronger. Closer. Although we admit in many ways we are still weak and fear often tries to come in and ruin our happiness. I guess you should say we're a work in progress.

The hardest lesson I've ever learned is to let go and not worry about the things that I can't control. The only one who has the power to watch over me and my family is the Lord. With each little victory and each little step, my faith continues to grow and my confidence continues to grow. I know that there were, and still are, so many people praying for me and that is the only way I was able to come through.

It would have been very easy for us to question God—why did I have cancer, why was he allowing Robin to become depressed and withdrawn?

What we've learned, though, is to keep our faith strong. Never let go of what we know is true, that with God's love we WILL persevere. Some people don't hold on to that belief, and that may work for them. But we choose to accept the promises God has given us. And, it IS a choice.

Life is what we make it. Our happiness depends on US. The decisions we make, how we react to what life gives us, those are choices WE make.

IT'S ABOUT SHARING EXPERIENCES

Seeing things differently

You are about to read the innermost thoughts of several young women across America who have watched their mothers battle breast cancer.

It was a simple idea—send an announcement out to my mom's Internet writing groups asking if they had a personal experience, or friends or family, with a mother who had breast cancer.

The response was overwhelming, and soon we were sending questionnaires to those willing to participate about how their moms' breast cancer affected their life.

They were all given the same questions. But their answers reveal that their cancer experience affected them in many different ways.

I know it helped ME to see what they went through, how they felt, and where they are now. I hope it helps you too!

And, to Megan, Ana, Dana, Laura, Sarah, Lauren, and Lindsay, I thank them for their candor. I appreciate their compassion for helping others through their words. And, I understand that their lives were changed the day cancer became a part of them. The battle is not won overnight—only fought one day at a time.

Because my mom didn't want to ask anyone to do something that she wouldn't ask of her own family, she asked me and my brother, Matt, to complete the questionnaire too. My mom put our answers into an interview format. Here goes...

Robin's Experience

Robin was 15 when her mom was diagnosed with breast cancer. Her first reaction was no reaction at all. She just said "Okay," walked out of the room, and didn't give it much thought.

"I was scared to even think about it."

She said that at the time she didn't turn to anyone for support because talking about it wasn't an option for her.

"I had so many mixed emotions and verbalized them to no one. I don't think I even really talked to my mom about it until a year or two later. I know that sounds awful, but I would have been beside myself. I was like that on the inside, I just didn't let it out."

Robin doesn't remember how long her mom's diagnosis and treatment stage lasted. There were a couple of biopsies and the mastectomy. Then smaller surgeries for reconstruction. But the ordeal completely changed the way Robin interacted with her family and friends.

"I was very withdrawn from my family, always afraid that someone would want to talk to me about it. I was content being by myself in my room.

"I remember one time in particular that my grandmother called and wanted my mom and me to come to a church function for ladies only. I sat on the bathroom floor pretending to be sick at my stomach until my mom came to see if I was ready to leave. I'm not sure how convinced she really was, but she left me there alone, which is what I wanted.

"After that I continued to cut off communication with my best friend, whom I had known since I was nine-years old. She would call, wanting to go to the mall or to the movies. But I always made something up or didn't return her calls. It came to where I was completely avoiding her."

Robin admits that she had a strong support group of family and friends available, but she didn't want their help.

"I think I received the support and guidance that I would allow. I didn't really reach out for a lot of that, but when I seldom did, family was always there.

"Although people asking me if I was okay was one of the things I hated the most. That question made me stop and think that no, I was not okay. But if you tell someone you're not okay, follow-up questions come and I did NOT want that."

Robin doesn't feel she was prepared for the affects her mom's cancer had on her. But doesn't think anyone can be.

"I really don't know if anyone prepared my mom for the affect it would have on HER either, though. I guess no one can tell you the affect something of that magnitude is going to have. How could anyone have possibly known this is what would happen to me?

After some time had passed, Robin stresses that she did eventually turn to someone for help.

"I really didn't have any support from outside the family. I didn't keep in touch with anyone from school, except one. I believe she was there to serve as a distraction, which is what I needed some of the times. Just to act like a kid for a while, giggle about silly things, and not feel depressed was a wonderful thing.

"Anyway, the greatest source of support and comfort has always been my family, my Nanny and Pappaw (my grandparents). My mom has always been my best friend, but there is just something about going to my grandparent's and having them comfort me. That's who I turned to. Those are some of the times in my life when I have felt so loved and protected."

Robin is very candid about how her mom's cancer has changed her life.

"My mom's battle with breast cancer had such an affect on me, both physically and emotionally, and that will always be with me.

"Once everything started to sink in, I was completely terrified of losing her. And eleven years later, I STILL AM.

"The physical affects didn't surface until I was about sixteen or probably closer to seventeen. I had so much emotion, feelings that I wanted to express, nervousness, panic attacks, and worry, that I literally worried myself sick. I mean sick to my stomach. Such panic would set in and I would be crying so hard that I was causing myself throw up.

"Of course after that happened a few times, I started panicking that I would do that in front of someone. That, in itself, would cause enough of a panic or anxiety attack, that I would end up getting sick just at the thought of everything.

"I got to where I wanted to stay in my room, that's the only place that I felt okay and I could relax.

"Even today, those attacks will still sneak up on me every once in a while, but back then they were pretty consistent and were amazingly unbearable until I was a little over eighteen and went to the doctor for the first time about it.

"I am still on medications for depression and have been under a doctor's care for the last eight years. The medicine improves my quality of life, equalizes the screwed up chemicals my brain creates, and helps me cope. Some people say anti-depressants mask problems and that there is no such thing as chemical imbalance. But I can't worry about what some people say. I just know how I was then and how I am now.

"I truly believe that family, faith, and yes, even doctors, are what helped me battle what I feel will be life-long affects of a cancer experience."

Even though things are easier now, and she has gotten past the hardest parts, Robin does have regrets. She definitely wishes she had done things differently.

"Obviously, I hope I never have this to go through again, but I would have spent so much more time with my mom. Not being there for her at that time in her life is the biggest regret I have as an adult. I can't believe that I left her there alone with just our dog and cat.

"She had drains that she would have to take care of on her own. I was just a selfish kid and me not being sad or having to think about losing my Mom was more important to me than helping her get through one of the toughest periods in her life."

As for advice to others who have a mother with a serious illness, this is what Robin says:

"I don't know if I SHOULD give any advice to other teens going through a similar situation. It kind of sounds like I didn't make it so great.

"But, the one thing I would say is GET THROUGH IT. However it is you need to cope, do it! Whether it's becoming a hermit like I did

and not talking about it or getting counseling, talking to people
at church, or starting your own
group with people that you know
are going through the same thing.
Getting through it is the only
goal, in my opinion. Whatever that
takes.

"No one can tell you how you
should cope with something. Just
let your mom know how much you appreciate and love her. There are
so many people that aren't as
lucky and blessed as I am, my
mommy is still here.

"I am so thankful for everything I went through because it
made me who I am today. Stronger,
more appreciative of everything
that I have, and closer with my
family. I have more faith, knowing
that I can overcome something like
this. Sometimes you just need to
step out in faith and know that
your loved ones will be there. You
don't have to do everything on
your own, and you won't be burden-
ing the people who love you, by
asking for their support and love.

Matt's Experience
Matt's eighteenth birthday was

spent alone at home, while his mom was in the hospital recovering from her mastectomy and reconstruction. And, even with the attention focused on her, he didn't feel left out. This is how he answered when asked if his needs were ever ignored:

"I'm pretty self-sufficient and wouldn't have noticed if anyone was paying less attention to me unless it was monumental...and that wasn't the case."

It's hard to know if his reactions are typical to guys in general, or just to him, but all his answers are very straightforward.

When finding out about his mom's cancer, his first reaction wasn't fear, anger, OR helplessness.

"I wasn't that worried. I guess because Mom told me that she detected it early enough and the doctors informed her that a full recovery was probable."

He didn't talk about the cancer to anyone outside the family, and would go to his sister and mom if he needed to talk about his feelings. His mom, he says, was his greatest source of support and comfort.

"My mom came to me and told me about her biopsy results; that she had cancer. And, at the same time, she told me the exact state of things. I saw it as something that was going to be okay," Matt said. "So, while I wasn't prepared for what we might go through as a family, I just looked to the doctor's prognosis for guidance."

Matt admits he came through the cancer experience without the lasting emotional effects his sister suffered. And, although he was lucky, he still says there are things he would do differently.

"Well, I know my mom thought at one point that I was completely indifferent to her ordeal. My trust in her, in the doctors, and that everything would be fine gave a perception that I didn't care too much about things. So, I think if I had to do it all over again, I would reiterate and reassure her more often. Because my thoughts were always on her and her situation."

As to advice he'd give others facing the same situation, Matt says, "Do your homework and use the Internet and doctor's advise to get 100% informed on what is happening.

"Don't lie to yourself and try to sugar coat things. If it's bad, be prepared for it and get everyone up to date on the situation."

He also adds, "Be sure you let your mom know you're going through it with her. Even if she is optimistic and has a good prognosis, you want her to know you care about her.

"The appearance of not caring was hard for our family, but is now a non-issue, since we sat down and talked about it."

Reflections from The Past
Megan, Ana, Dana, Laura, Sarah

MEGAN
Megan was sixteen years old when her mom was diagnosed with cancer. Both her parents told her about it. Her first reaction was fear. She accepted the diagnosis, but didn't really talk to anyone about it.

It took about a year to get from the diagnosis to the end of treatment, with Megan helping care

for her mom about twenty five percent of the time. And, although
she says it definitely affected
the way she interacted with
friends and family, she was able
to deal with it because of her
circle of support. Now, years
later, she is proud to say she has
never required a doctor's care or
medicine for depression. She read
books and found resources on the
Internet to answer her questions.

Megan says her advice to other
girls/young women who have a
mother with a serious illness is,
"Be open about it. Make sure your
mom keeps a positive attitude. And
find people you can talk to. Don't
be afraid to take support."

The only thing she would've
done differently is to have been
more open with her sister.

ANA

Ana was sixteen years old when
her mom was diagnosed. "I remember
my mom went for a mammogram, her
first one ever, I believe, and she
said they found a lump, but it
was probably just a cyst, and not
to worry. So I didn't."

Ana says after the biopsy and

additional tests, her mom and dad sat her down and told her that her mom was going to have a mastectomy. That was that.

Ana admits her first reaction was fear, anger and helplessness. And then the denial took over. She never really talked to anyone, even her best friend, about how she was feeling.

From the time of diagnosis, to the end of treatment, it was about a year. When I asked Ana if she had been responsible for taking part in her mother's care, this is what she told me.

"I tried to be helpful, but my dad was taking care of her, and it seemed like she really didn't even want my help, so I kinda just stayed away."

Ana admits that the ordeal didn't affect her relationship with her friends and family, but it definitely had an emotional affect on HER. She needed support and guidance but confides she didn't ask for it. She just tried to occupy her life with other things.

She wasn't prepared for the emotional toll it would take on

her. And she continues to suffer with anxiety and depression, but is not under a doctor's care.

If she could change the way she handled anything, it would be, "I would have tried to talk to my mother about her condition more...instead of just keeping it to myself."

Ana, years later, still feels the effects of her mom's cancer. These are her closing thoughts:

"At the time my mother was diagnosed and had surgery, I never thought about getting breast cancer...it is only now, five years later, that I think of it constantly.

"I'm always thinking I've found a lump in my breasts. Then I go to the gynecologist, where she tells me it's nothing and not to worry. But, I'm paranoid. Almost every woman on my mother's side of the family has had some type of cancer.

"And when my friend's mom died of breast cancer last year, that definitely triggered a lot of fear again. Wondering if my mother would get cancer in her other breast, if it would come back."

"I live with that fear almost every day."

DANA

Dana was thirteen years old when her mom was diagnosed with cancer. No one prepared her or counseled with her about what to expect. Her mom just explained that she had cancer and would need surgery.

And, although she accepted and understood the diagnosis and the treatment, her initial reaction to the news was fear and confusion.

Dana's mom and her best friend wanted to offer support, but they couldn't relate to what Dana was going through. So, basically, she didn't talk to anyone about what she really felt. Just told people the facts about it.

Dana tells me that she didn't turn to the Internet to search for answers. But, she did read the things her mom would find and give to her.

While Dana says she wouldn't really do anything differently, if she had it to do over again, she does have some advice for other girls going through this.

"It's okay to ask for help every once in a while. That was a hard lesson for me, and my mom, to learn."

LAURA

Laura was fifteen years old when her mom was diagnosed with cancer. She is one of the ones who appeared to manage very well at the time, but who found that issues connected came back later, in college.

Her initial reaction to the news was numbness. And the appearance of acceptance.

"My father came to school to tell me the news. They paged me to the office and my father told me, although now I can't remember at all what he said.

"Then I went to the lunchroom, where lunch was underway and told a number of my friends." But she didn't discuss her feelings with them.

Throughout the year of her mother's treatment, Laura spent about twenty-five percent of her time caring for her mother and the additional household chores she inherited. Her father was too overwhelmed with his own sadness to offer support, though he did learn to cook.

When asked who provided emotional support, Laura said, "Church folks were very supportive. But, I don't remember there being a lot of support from within the family. Who had the time for that? However, this is where relatives, adult friends, and godparents can and SHOULD really step up to the plate for the kids going through this.

"It's natural to focus a lot on the sick person. But, I think that our basic needs were taken care of by family and friends. Although I'm sure that certain things went by the wayside. I remember having trouble finding concentrated time to study."

Next, I asked Laura if the cancer had affected her relationships with her friends, or if it kept her from doing normal 'teen-age' things. And how/if it affected her emotional well-being as she got older.

"Relationships affected? Yes. Memorably. I got taken out to the homecoming dance by a friend who told me at the dance that it was a mercy date. He felt sorry for me. That was pretty crushing. In retrospect, most of my friends didn't really know what to make of it either.

"As far as my emotional wellbeing, yes, I think the experience affected me. It's hard to quantify, though. It's hard to say how feeling/being entirely irrelevant to one's family for a certain chunk of time affects one.

"Any problems really arose later, in college. I had a lot of trouble in college relating on a normal level to my parents; always felt like I couldn't report anything that might upset them, all the while I was engaging in self-destructive behaviors that they would have disapproved of though, nothing really scary dangerous. We're talking about drinking and smoking here.

"I did have terrible migraine headaches during a period of about a year when I was nineteen, which I think probably betokened depression which I just kind of snapped out of on my own around the beginning of junior year. I've always been kind of self-sufficient that way, but it probably would have helped to see a therapist to work out some of the issues. On the other hand, how much is teen angst and how much is cancer? It's impossible to separate them."

As far as resources, Laura tells me the Internet wasn't yet a useful tool when she went through this years ago, but she followed the news on cancer and she read "When Bad things Happen to Good People."

When I asked Laura what, in hindsight, she would've done differently, she couldn't think of much.

"I might try to reach out more for help, but honestly, there's not so much you can do. Cancer is the ultimate "not about you" thing, isn't it?"

And, here's Laura's advice for everyone with a mother who is facing illness.

"I'd say the most important thing is to remember that your parents love is what got you here, and it is the same love that makes them both, but especially your dad, crazy with grief and fear.

"Sometimes they can't help but take it out on the people around them. So, to a certain extent, you have to just grit your teeth through the irritability.

"But if it gets really bad, you should definitely talk to a teacher or a rabbi/priest/minister or adult friend who can maybe help to give you an outlet and a break.

"And remember: it's these challenges that make you into a kid who knows a lot more about the real meaning of love and life than most people are privileged to learn so young. It can make you a more compassionate person than most."

SARAH

Let me start Sarah's section by saying that she is the sister of Laura, above. Their answers were sent in independent of the other. It's interesting to see how different their accounts are.

"I am assuming that Mom put you in contact with my older sister, Laura. I think she had a harder time, since she was a bit older than me, and therefore more was expected of her. However, it's been so long since Mom had cancer that some of your questions are quite hard for me to answer.

"I know that her cancer changed all of us in the family, and I am sure that we all had 'ugly' moments (or even months), but in the end, we all came out fine, still loving one another."

Sarah was eleven years old when her mom was diagnosed with cancer. Her first reaction was uncertainty. And, since she didn't understand the seriousness of the diagnosis, she basically took what she was told at face value.

Sarah doesn't remember discussing her feelings with anyone. Although she's sure that she talked to her mom and dad about the surgery and the chemo, and no doubt, talked to her older sister about it too, she doesn't think her feelings were discussed.

"Generally I was prone to worry, which is why I think that Mom and Dad glossed over the more serious aspects of the cancer diagnosis. Although I don't remember sleepless nights, I am sure that I did worry about what would happen should Mom not get better."

The time of her mother's cancer battle, diagnosis and treatment, lasted about nine months. Sarah wasn't really needed for tending to her mom's needs, specifically, but was given extra household duties such as laundry, dishes, cleaning/picking up, making dinner, and making her own lunches for school. But she feels this made her much more self-sufficient than most other kids her age.

"It's hard for me to remember, and I really only have a few memories of it...but I remember the week we ate seven layered salad every night. This was after Mom had had the initial surgery, and the women in the volunteer group at our church were organizing dinner for us every other night. I guess seven layered salad must have been on everyone's minds. I just remember that we joked that when one gets cancer, one must eat seven-layered salad. Morbid, I know, but I guess that's how we dealt with some of the fear.

"And I remember the day my father flew into a rage after my mother reported that my sister had not been helpful to her. This was after one of Mom's chemo sessions, and Dad had to work, so we were supposed to be helpful and bring food, water, and generally fetch things for Mom. His reaction scared me more than anything else that happened, because I had never seen my father angry before. It was at this point, that I realized things were more serious than they seemed."

Sarah says she turned to her older sister, Laura, who provided the greatest amount of support in her family. And that her dog provided comfort.

"I'm not sure this counts, but I do remember snuggling up with our dog a lot and talking to her."

If Sarah could've changed anything, she would have been more helpful to her mom, understanding now the pain of the surgery and the exhaustion that the chemo caused. She also would have been more appreciative of the time they spent together.

Her advice to others who have a mom with a serious illness: "Find an ally in a sibling or in a friend so that you can feel comfortable talking to someone about what's going on. Don't be afraid to let your mother know that you are worried or scared. Don't try to shoulder all of mom's duties. Don't try to become your family's mom."

Sarah says she remembers how different her mom seemed after the surgery. Her "life's too short to deal with this sh*t" attitude. This was a great life lesson that I was able to internalize at a young age.

Day by Day
Lauren, Lindsay

At the time of their inter- view, these two sisters had just gone through their mother's cancer battle. She had just completed six months of chemotherapy. We espe- cially appreciate their strength and willingness to discuss their feelings while their pain and fears were still fresh.

LAUREN
Lauren was twelve when her mom was diagnosed with cancer. She is the younger of the two sisters. Her initial reaction was fear, an-

ger, and sadness, and she dealt with it by denial.

She says her mom was the one who told her, and she just said she had cancer.

Lauren credits her mom and dad as her greatest source of support within the family. Her best friend, as the greatest support outside the family. And a strong faith in God as the source of comfort and courage.

No one really prepared Lauren for the effect her mom's cancer would have on her. But she adds that it never kept her from doing things she wanted to do, even though she was called on to take care of additional household duties.

"I was sad a lot of times," Lauren admits. "But not always. I should have helped my mom more than I did, though."

As for comments or advice she'd like to share with other girls who have a mom with a serious illness, she says, "Pray...Pray hard. There is nothing greater than God's love and care."

LINDSAY

Lindsay was fourteen years old when her mom was diagnosed with cancer. And, like her sister, her initial reaction was fear, anger, and helplessness.

"I just kept praying that it was a dream, and that I'd wake up and everything would be okay again."

And, while she tells me that she initially turned to a friend to talk about her feelings, Lindsay says her greatest source of support and comfort within her family was her sister, Lauren.

"My sister probably helped me the most. Since we're so close we really stuck together and talked about things a lot to try to help each other out.

"Outside my family, the greatest source of support came from my best friend's mom, Jeanne. She's a counselor, and she was so supportive. I remember her being there the night we found out.

"We were all sitting in our living room, watching a parade on TV. My mom got a call and started writing things down, information. I knew she had it then. We all started crying, but Mom and Dad promised us that we would be okay.

"That's when Jeanne took us to McDonald's. It's kind of strange, but we just sat in the car and talked through a lot. She let us cry on her shoulder. I love her for that."

I asked Lindsay if anyone prepared her for the effect her mom's cancer would have on her.

"I had no idea that is was going to be as hard as it was."

Lindsay admits she would occasionally read a story about cancer, but said she didn't go to the Internet for information, because she was already scared out of her mind and didn't want to learn more than she already knew.

As far as the cancer experience changing the relationships she had with friends and family, Lindsay says, "The experience affected me. It helped me become closer with several people in my life because of their help, support, and positive influence on my life.

"It also made me realize how fortunate we were. At first I was very upset and wondered why it had to happen to us. But, then, I told myself I was thankful everyone else was healthy in our family, and that her cancer could be treated."

My next question to Lindsay was if she ever felt she missed out on anything while everyone was taking care of her mom?

"Mom was, and should have been, the main focus during the majority of the six months of her treatment. However, when we went on a family vacation to Florida (something we do every year) it wasn't any fun with Mom being sick. Sometimes people would ask me to go do something, but I was just too down."

Talking to the young girls who may have still been adjusting to their emotions, I was concerned they might not be up to answering questions. So I always asked how talking about it made them feel.

"I don't mind talking about it," Lindsay said. "It had a major impact on my life, and it hurt very badly when our family was going through it. But we made it through. And, if anyone ever needed advice, or wanted to talk about it, I would definitely be open to that."

Here is some of the advice Lindsay would give to them.

"I would just say that I know it's difficult, and you're going to be asking 'WHY' all the time. It's an incredibly hard fact to face. But the only thing that kept me going was my faith. I was constantly praying. Without God's help I would not have made it.

"What also helped me was the support of my friends. One thing I did wrong was to *not* express my feelings. I was either too afraid that I would lose it and have a breakdown in front of them, or that they wouldn't understand. But I think the most important thing is to let your close friends know how you are feeling, so they can help you in anyway needed.

"Just talk to people. Get it out. And pray."

Author's note: All the above recollections were taken from answers on the questionnaires. Sometimes the comments were taken in part, other times a word or two may have been added to create a paragraph, or for grammatical correctness. However, the integrity of the answers were not altered.

IT'S ABOUT PROFESSIONALS©

Teens and Cancer in the Family©
by Nancee Biank

Being diagnosed with breast cancer can be a terrifying experience. You are catapulted into a world of information-seeking and decision-making that brings with it uncertainty and more questions than answers. Being a single parent and mother of two only complicates the diagnosis. How do I tell the children? What do I tell them? What will they think? Who will help me? These are just a few of the questions that run through the mind of a mother. Are you going to die? is always a question that is on the mind of every child, even if it never gets asked.

As a therapist who has worked with over 700 children and adolescents who have a family member with cancer, it has been my job to help families ferret through all

116

of the confusion and chaos that can arise at the time of a diagnosis and through the treatment. After ten years of helping families I can honestly say there is no one right way to tell your children, extended family, or friends about your diagnosis. There are some things that we recommend, however, but first and foremost remember you know your children better than anyone, so check your gut before you speak.

In general it is recommended that you sit down with your children once you have all of the information and have made a decision on the course of treatment. Prior to that time you really don't have enough definitive information to share and can just create more anxiety by sharing all of the options. If you are required to have a second mammogram or a CAT scan early on, you can honestly say: "Mom has to get some tests or mom has a doctor appointment," if you feel the need to explain your absences. If a biopsy is required, again a short explanation will suffice. Mom has a little lump on her breast that Dr Sxxxxx is going to remove and test for the possibility of disease. I will be home later today and might be a little sore, but I will be fine in a few days.

It is once the results of the biopsy are given and a course of action has been chosen that it's time to talk with the children. Prior to this, remember that children and adolescents are very astute. They listen behind closed doors, while you are talking on the telephone, and while you are in conversation with Aunt Mary or Uncle Ed, so BE DISCREET.

When talking with children it is important to give honest but age appropriate information. You would not go into the same details with a six year old as you would with a sixteen year old. For the younger crowd it is important to say mom has been diagnosed with cancer (call it by name) and talk about what it is and what the doctors are going to do. Such as: "Breast cancer is a disease that changes some of the cells in mommy's body. These cells can be hurtful to the rest of my body so the doctor wants to get rid of them. The way we get rid of them is by: cutting out the ones that the doctor can see, giving mom some medicine for the ones that might be left-it is called chemotherapy, and then to make sure there are no more cancer cells; giving mommy something called radiation. Radiation is a special x-ray. It uses the same process as when you get pictures taken of your teeth to see if you have any cavities. The difference is that radiation can be done on a very tiny specific area that can help get rid of cancer because it is stronger than what is used to take pictures of your teeth."

Another important piece of information to share is how you will feel and the possible loss of your hair. You can tell young children that the medicine that the doctor is going to give you may make you tired and a little sick to your stomach so you may need to rest more. You should also add the possibility of hair loss. Some treatments don't result in hair loss but most do. If your cancer treatment is one that does, it is imperative to prepare the children. Young and school age children seem to be more bothered by hair loss than middle school or teenage children. Although teenagers may be more vocal about asking you to put on a scarf or keep on your wig if their friends are around. They are also game for participating in a party where you shave your head or growing their own hair for a cause such as "Locks of Love" an organization that makes wigs for pediatric cancer patients. In any event tell the children that your hair will fall out and that means your eyelashes as well.

When breaking the news, allow time for questions. Some children may have none that they will ask right away, while others may ask a myriad of what you may think are senseless questions. Answer them all as honestly as possible. As stated earlier, the biggest question that is on everyone's mind is: "Are you going to die?" A child or teen may be too scared or embarrassed to ask the question, but trust me, at some level they are thinking it. It is better to address it head on rather than skirt around an answer. When originally telling the children, the answer to the question would be something like this: "Right now I do not believe that I am going to die from my cancer. The doctors and mom have met and decided on the best treatment for my type of cancer. They promised me they will do everything they can to make sure I get the best treatment. I promise you that I will do everything in my power to follow their instructions and take all of my medicine. What I need you to do during this time is be a part of my Cancer Support Team and do the things that you should do-your chores, homework, play with friends, and promise me that we will take the time to talk about whatever is on your mind. Deal? Deal! If anything changes you will be the first to know, but for now lets continue to be a family as much as we can and just help each other out when we need it."

If there are tears during this talk it is okay. Children need to know that it is okay to feel mad, sad, and bad when they hear about a diagnosis of cancer in a family member. For other questions, answer them as honestly as possible or simply state: "I don't know the answer to that question; it is a good question, so maybe we can find out the answer together."

This brings us to the subject of the Internet and your teenager. Don't be surprised if they are busy gathering their own information. This can be problematic, because not all websites are accurate and reliable. However there are some websites that are, and there is even an online support group available for teens that have a parent with cancer.

Actions and reactions

When a parent is diagnosed with breast cancer there are several reactions that can occur. I have worked with teenage boys who have retreated to their bedrooms not to come out until they have been involved in a support group and connected with others experiencing the same feelings. There have been teenage girls who have been called home from college to be by their mother's side throughout the entire experience.

Others have gone to school, stayed out late and begun acting out in ways so atypical to their personhood that parents have been shocked. Still others keep their routine as much as possible and help out at home when they can. All of these reactions are within the range of normal for when a parent has cancer. How they are handled by the family and professionals is what is different.

Adolescents are more aware and most affected by the diagnosis because they are in a stage of development where they should begin separating and individuating from the family.

When a parent is diagnosed, especially a single mother, the children can be called upon to become a "partner" to that parent. This can be a difficult role. The child wants to participate and help as much as possible but it can interfere with their growth and development.

In the case of the teen that was called home from college to be with her mother, taking her to chemotherapy and doctor appointments, her reaction was life changing. After her mother's recovery, she never returned to school, met a man and went to live in another state. If the family had given more thought to the needs of the mom and worked as a team things may have turned out differently for their daughter.

The importance of developing a CANCER SUPPORT TEAM or CaST is paramount. When you are diagnosed with cancer there are many people who want to help. This is the time to LET THEM. Make a list of each task that needs to be done, no matter how small. Decide which person is best for each task and ask them to help out. They will be happy to help, and you will be relieved of a lot of stress.

In a single parent family this can be even more necessary than in a two parent family. Children automatically want to help and should participate some, but when the burden falls on one child or one child instinctively takes on all of the tasks, stop and reassess. The results can be damaging as was shown by the experience of

Cindy's daughter. Although years
after there are no regrets, the
journey could have been smoother
if a few precautions were taken.
Children are still children no
matter how old they are, when
their parent is sick. Find another
adult, a sister, a close friend,
or another family member to be the
co-anchor for the family during
this difficult time.

Communication/Non-Communication

Teens typically don't communi-
cate routinely with their parents
while they are busy mastering this
stage of development called sepa-
ration-individuation. It is their
task to test out their parents'
values and ideas by formulating
their own. After some time they
usually come around to integrating
the family values into what is
best for their generation.

When there is a diagnosis of
cancer, adolescents are called
back into the family system and
asked to resume their family role
or as mentioned, take on new helping behaviors. When this occurs,
the last bastion of remaining an

individual may be to keep their thoughts and concerns to themselves. Parents may constantly ask: "What are you thinking?" "Do you have any questions?" or state: "You are not talking with me? What are you hiding?" Your teen may leave the house every chance they get when you would appreciate their company. They may even start fights just to see if you can rise to the occasion and respond.

The answer to all of this is to HOLD ON TIGHT. When there is a diagnosis of cancer, everyone reacts and works at getting the family system back to its state of equilibrium that was comfortable prior to the diagnosis. The problem is the effects of cancer can last 3-5 years, and there is a new normal that becomes established. Life is not the same as before. When children and adolescents act out, they are testing your parenting. Can you still be there for them? Will you still get angry at what mattered before? Can you contain them? Maintain the family rules as much as possible. That means the same curfew, the same rules about chores, and the same rules about school and homework. The more the structure of the family remains close to pre-diagnosis the better the family will function.

If there is cancer support centers near your home, check on whether they have a support group for your children and/or adolescent. It can give your children a place to address their concerns and an opportunity to be with other children or teens that are going through a similar situation. Teens will not want to attend but ask them to try it for three sessions and once they attend they may be pleasantly surprised at the level of camaraderie and identification they feel with the group. Support groups are not for everyone, but I have personally experienced 700 children and adolescents who think that they were helpful during their family journey through cancer.

Moving forward

Since cancer can last fifty percent of the life of a ten year old or thirty percent of the life of a fifteen year old, for the child, life has essentially changed as they knew it. Everyone must adjust to a "new normal." There is a roller coaster effect that families talk about. Just as we are getting ready to resume our lives, there is a doctor appointment that reminds us mom had cancer.

"What will be the results of the 3, 6, or 12 month check-up, or the yearly follow-up after that? Will it come back? What will happen if it does? Who will take care of me? How will I handle telling my children this time?" All of these questions are ever present, only to arise if the test results bring suspicion. How does a family move forward during this time?

'One day at a time' is a cliché but one that works when there is a diagnosis of cancer. Learning to live in the moment and appreciating each day are two lessons that cancer can teach us—not easily, but they can be learned. Practicing meditation and relaxation as a family can be helpful in order to quell any anxiety and "what-ifs" that may arise. *(Biank has a CD useful for teaching relaxation to children and another for adolescents.)*

Coming together as a family to deal with the questions that will present themselves can also be helpful. Keeping a sense of humor during and after the journey is imperative. Laughter is good for the soul and also produces endorphins that make us feel better.

As the journey continues take time to do the things that you and your family enjoy so that memories are built and time together is not wasted.

IT'S ABOUT RESOURCES

Information is power. So Robin and I have searched the Internet, asked friends, talked to counselors, and compiled a list of all the resources they referred us to.

Books...

(* indicates author favorites— Cindy read these titles during her own cancer battle)

➢ ***Breast Cancer for Dummies*** - by Ronit Elk, Monica Morrow

If you or someone you love has been diagnosed with breast cancer, you're probably confused, afraid, shocked, or even angry. Or you may be all of the above. Let this book become your trusted manual. Discover more about the cancer, explore treatment options, find ways to make this part of your life

easier. Let shared experiences
serve as your knowledgeable guide
and anchor to help you make wise
and confident choices.

Think of breast cancer as a
journey and this book as your
roadmap. Have you already been diagnosed? In that case, this book
can help you explore these important truths:

• Breast cancer is not a death
sentence. Most women diagnosed
with early stage breast cancer can
look forward to enjoying a
healthy, full life.

• Not only are you unique as a
person, but so, too, is your particular form of cancer, your
treatment options, and your prognosis.

• Every day more is discovered
about how to prevent, detect earlier, and more effectively treat
breast cancer.

• You are not alone. More than
two million women in the United
States today are breast cancer
survivors. Thousands of groups and
programs across the country offer
support, and chances are, one is
close to your neighborhood.

This book can help you feel like you have a sister who's a doctor, a sister who tells you what to expect every step of the way, who gives you the best advice she can, and guides you along the way. (Of course, there is absolutely no replacement for advice about *you* from your own doctor.) You'll feel empowered to know and understand what's going on in your body, so that you can become a part of your own treatment team and make decisions along with your doctors and your family. (an Amazon.com review)

➢ ***Cancer: 50 Essential Things to Do**** - by Greg Anderson, O. Carl Simonton (Foreword)

This definitive guide, revised and updated with over 25% new material, empowers cancer patients and their loved ones to move beyond their disease. Greg Anderson, a cancer survivor, has designed this book for the recently diagnosed, those with recurring symptoms, and those who are well but have a lingering fear that the disease may strike again.

Informative and inspiring, *Cancer: 50 Essential Things to Do* goes hand-in-hand with the patient's medical treatment and is an invaluable roadmap to recovery. Filled with practical, healing "action steps" that have been used by thousands of cancer survivors, the revised edition also contains important new information, including recently approved medical treatment options, updated cancer research, and Internet resources-geared toward making sense of the fast-changing world of cancer treatment and recovery. (an Amazon.com review)

➤ *Living Beyond Breast Cancer: A Survivor's Guide for When Treatment Ends and the Rest of Your Life Begins* - *by Marisa Weiss, Ellen Weiss*

If you are one of the 2.6 million women in the U.S. living beyond breast cancer, these may be some of the questions troubling you. You've been through diagnosis and treatment; now you're ready to move from "I have breast cancer" back to "I am leading a normal life." *Living Beyond Breast Cancer* will help you understand and manage the tough issues you face as you go on beyond treatment, and well into the future.

You'll learn how to become as healthy as possible for as long as possible by eating right, managing your weight, and finding an exercise program that works with your lifestyle. You'll find out what to do if you've got to stop taking hormones or want to start. You may also need advice on achieving intimacy and having a baby. You'll also find invaluable guidance on growing older and navigating troubling symptoms of menopause, particularly when they're brought on by chemotherapy or tamoxifen or by stopping hormone replacement therapy. A normal life includes dealing with job and health care issues and wills. So you'll find in-depth information on these subjects too.

You're a survivor, and you've got a future. This empathetic book, filled with comprehensive medical information, practical advice, and the voices of survivors who have lived through everything

you're going through, will help
you celebrate your second chance
at living beyond breast cancer.
(an Amazon.com review)

➢ *The Breast Cancer Survival Man-*
   ual, Third Edition : A Step-by-
   Step Guide for the Woman With
   Newly Diagnosed Breast Cancer -
   by John Link, et al:

   In a valuable guide for women
who have just been diagnosed with
breast cancer, Dr. John Link helps
sort through the confusion and the
fear, by explaining such things as
how to get a second opinion and
how to understand a pathology report.
   Particularly valuable is Link's
step-by-step description of how
breast cancer is characterized, or
staged, according to tumor size,
hormone receptors, and other factors and how that affects prognosis. As a breast cancer specialist
at Long Beach and Orange Coast Memorial hospitals in Southern Cali-
fornia, Link knows the medical
jargon and what it means. Although
his writing style is at times a
bit jargony and difficult to read,

a breast cancer patient will willingly read and reread every word. The book also includes useful chapters on diet, exercise, herbs, and vitamins; managing the side effects of treatment; healing's mind-body connection; and organizing medical records and keeping a personal journal or log.

Ending on an encouraging note, Link writes, "You should know that most women today are cured of breast cancer. They undergo treatment, become survivors, and go on with their lives. But having breast cancer is certainly a wake-up call to many and may be for you. Life now has added uncertainty." This step-by-step manual helps you navigate the uncertainty and become a survivor, both physically and psychologically. (*an Amazon.com review.*)

➢ *The Cancer Dictionary* – by Roberta Altman, Michael Sarg

The Cancer Dictionary is useful for brief definitions of terms and ready-reference questions, but those in need of more detailed information about specific cancers or treatments should consult other resources. (an Amazon.com review)

➢ ***The Complete Idiot's Guide to Living with Breast Cancer -***_by Sharon Sorenson, Suzanne Metger

Annually, about 185,000 women (and a few men) face the diagnosis of breast cancer, and the numbers are on the rise. If you're one of those diagnosed—or know somebody who is—you understand that fighting the disease is a down-and-dirty war with lots of skirmishes and full-blown battles on the way to victory. The good news is that at this moment over two million survivors—vibrant, active women making significant contributions to their families and communities—carry the victory flag.

How do we know about these folks? We're two of them. We're survivors who have been through the surgeries and through the treatments, and our battle scars have left us with a keen sense of empathy. We firmly believe that nobody should have to face breast cancer alone. Ever. So as we put words to paper, we visualized an in-print support group—messages from breast cancer survivors who shared their stories and offered the 20/20 vision of hindsight. Some have carried the victory flag for 20 years or more; others are still in the battlefield, reporting from the front lines. And trust us when we say that these front-line warriors fight with a courage and determination that have humbled us day after day.

If you've found yourself drafted in the war against breast cancer—or know someone who is—this book offers the support you need, from the first hint of a lump or suspicious mammogram through surgery and treatment and on to follow-up for the rest of your life.

In short, we'll be there to get you through all the battles, with hugs and cookies from home. May your battles be short and your victory sweet. (author's Amazon review)

➢ *Encyclopedia of Herbal Medicine: The Definitive Home Reference Guide to 550 Key Herbs with all their Uses as Remedies for Com-*

mon Ailments - by Andrew Cheval-
lier, Gillian Emerson-Roberts

Featuring more than 550 medicinal plants and the most current
scientific research, this volume
provides a comprehensive guide to
healing with the world's oldest
form of medicine. A unique photo-
graphic index profiles over 550
plants, with detailed information
on habitat and cultivation, parts
used, active constituents, therapeutic properties, and traditional
and current uses.

A special section profiles 100
of the most common plants, featuring herbal preparations and recom-
mendations for self-treatment.
Guidelines on growing, harvesting,
and storing medicinal plants also
demonstrate making remedies for
home use. In addition, accessible
text offers fascinating insight
into the chemistry of plants and
their healing properties, explaining how and why they work as medi-
cines within the body. The major
herbal traditions of different
cultures—Europe, India, China, Af-
rica, Australia, and the Americas—
are vividly described. A review of

herbs from a historical perspective reveals the connection between medicinal herbs and cultural beliefs toward healing. Offering extensive coverage of all that herbs are—from cultural traditions to chemical components to self-treatments for common ailments—this Encyclopedia of Herbal Medicine is the ultimate reference for anyone interested in exploring the healing benefits of medicinal plants.

➢ *The Race Is Run One Step at a Time: Every Woman's Guide to Taking Charge of Breast Cancer & My Personal Story** - by Nancy G. Brinker, Catherine McEvilly Harris

Nancy Brinker's book is not intended for women alone, but for everyone. Breast cancer touches the lives of all of us. This important volume gives women, and the men and children who care for them, a starting point – a compass with which they can begin their race to obtain information. (excerpt from the introduction)

➢ ***The Victoria's Secret Catalog Never Stops Coming : And Other Lessons I Learned From Breast Cancer**** - by Jennie Nash

Touching and courageous, *The Victoria's Secret Catalog Never Stops Coming* blends the medical realities of breast cancer with the wise and thoughtful opinions of author Jennie Nash. Nash shares every step of her experience with breast cancer, from the first mammogram to the final reconstructive surgery, in a series of "lessons" that divide chapters into stories that are equally meaningful to survivors and their friends and families. While many of the individual stories are sad, taken as whole this is an ultimately positive book—Nash survives with her health and family intact and is spared harrowing chemo and further metastasizing.

Her lessons range from "bad news does less damage when it's shared" to "caregivers are human," and are illustrated with deeply personal stories of sobbing telephone messages, family arguments, and never-ending streams of frozen casseroles. The last lesson, "make the experience matter," revolves around Nash's first breast-cancer walk as a survivor, though it could just as easily revolve around the writing of this book, as it is sure to make a welcome difference in the lives of countless women. (an Amazon.com review)

Internet Support Groups & Websites...

American Cancer Society – Teens with Parents with Cancer: Want to meet other survivors in your area, find support, or offer support to current cancer patients? Explore the programs and services that give support to cancer patients, survivors, and loved ones.

www.acscsn.org/Talk_Shows_and_Stor ies/Caregiver/Teens_with_parents_w ith_cancer.html

Cancer 411: Cancer 411.org is the result of the combined efforts of two organizations, The Rory Foundation, and The Joyce Foundation. The mission of Cancer 411 is to put cancer patients, their families and doctors in touch with the critical information they need as quickly as possible.

www.cancer411.org/

Cycle of Hope: The Cycle of Hope shows how learning facts will lessen your fears, help you regain control of your emotions, and ultimately increase your chances of beating cancer.

Like a spinning wheel, fear of cancer can be thought of as a cycle of concerns that build upon each other. The Cycle of Fear represents fears encountered before and after diagnosis, during treatment, and in remission.

Fear is a healthy human emotion that deserves your attention and respect. However, don't let it control your emotions and decision-making abilities. Come to terms with your fears by understanding the problems you face. Knowledge generates hope.

www.cycleofhope.org/index.htm

Friends in Need: Friends in

Need is a site to give support for people involved with breast cancer. Maybe just a friendly hello or some words of comfort. Remember, you are never alone in times of need. Sharing similar experiences can be very rewarding and showing a little compassion can help people overcome many obstacles we may face from day to day!

http://www.friendsinneed.com/

Friends in Touch: Friends In Touch has won numerous awards for reaching out to other women around the world. They are not an organization...simply a group of friends who meet to help one another through their breast cancer journeys. They welcome any one who is a breast cancer patient, survivor, caregiver or friend.

Although the members of Friends In Touch help thousands each month, their greatest joy will be the day they can close down the website because breast cancer has been wiped off the map. Until then, they hope everyone who visits their website will find a wealth of hope, support and friendship...and then...pass it on.

http://groups.msn.com/FriendsInTou chCareTeam/

Gilda's Club: Gilda's Club is a special place where the focus is on *living* with cancer. And where men, women and children with any kind of cancer and their family members and friends can plan and build life-changing emotional and social support.

If you are a person with can-cer, family member or caring friend, we urge you to seek emo-tional and social support—it's as important as medical care. At Gilda's Club, where every member-ship is free-of-charge, a commu-nity of support is developed in which people of all ages with all kinds of cancer learn from one an-other how to live more fully.

www.gildasclub.org/

On Your Mind: On Your Mind is a website that provides information and support for teens and is run by a group of volunteer high school students from the Bay Area. With the help of a crisis center, they've put together various resources that they hope are helpful. You can check out their chat room, submit questions, and find resources. This project was started with the hope of providing a safe place to get information and to chat.

www.onyourmind.net/index.html

Susan G. Komen Breast Cancer Foundation: For more than 20 years, the Susan G. Komen Breast Cancer Foundation has been a global leader in the fight against breast cancer through its support of innovative research and community-based outreach programs. Working through a network of U.S. and international Affiliates and events like the Komen Race for the Cure®, the Komen Foundation is fighting to eradicate breast cancer as a life-threatening disease by funding research grants and supporting education, screening and treatment projects in communities around the world.

http://www.komen.org/

The Cancer Survivor Toolbox: The *Cancer Survival Toolbox*® is a free audio program designed to help cancer survivors and caregivers develop practical skills to deal with the diagnosis, treatment and challenges of cancer.

Use this web site to listen to Toolbox programs and access, resources to help you navigate the cancer survivorship experience.

www.cancersurvivaltoolbox.org/

Y-Me National Breast Cancer Organization: The mission of Y-ME National Breast Cancer Organization is to ensure, through information, empowerment and peer support, that no one faces breast cancer alone.

Thanks to the generosity of their donors, Y-ME and its network of Affiliates provide information and support to anyone touched by breast cancer. As originally envisioned by Y-ME's founders, all programs and services are available free-of-charge.

www.y-me.org/

Videos...

Bosom Buddies - Bosom Buddies, Inc. was founded by breast cancer survivors, Kay Alport and Kathy Kompare. Their goal is to provide information to help alleviate some of the fear and anxiety caused by the diagnosis of breast cancer. To that end, they have produced these videos.
° Woman To Woman: Breast Cancer and Reconstruction Options
° Partners in Hope: Families Talk About Breast Cancer
° Will Mom Be OK?: Families Talk About Breast Cancer

www.bosombuddies.org/index.html

Between Us - Between Us founder, and veteran filmmaker Mary Katzke was diagnosed with breast cancer in 1992, her only experience with the disease was watching her mother die from it nine years earlier. She searched in vain for a film which would show long term survivors who honestly portrayed

148

their experiences with the disease. She made a commitment that if she made her five-year anniversary, she would create the film she so desperately needed at the time.

Through the voices and faces of a wide cross-section of women of all ages, ethnic and economic backgrounds, we hear the inside story of facing treatment and recovering from a disease we all believed would lead to our demise. It is a very personal, intimate, and candid film which is finding a surprising number of additional and unexpected venues, from use as a sensitivity training tool for surgeons to a gift of hope for husbands and families.

- *Between Us* (1998/updated in 2001) which is the focus of this website is designed to offer survivor mentorship to women immediately upon diagnosis of breast cancer. Winner of Docker's Khakis for Women's Independent Vision Award.
- *Beyond Flowers* (2003) – Designed to provide practical information for the support team surrounding

a woman in crisis of diagnosis and treatment.

www.betweenus.org/index.html

Sutter Health Patient Education Videos - The Sutter Health network offers a complete array of services for cancer patients, including diagnosis, treatment, education and support.

Their cancer programs also collaborate and share expertise, with the goal of improving care for all cancer patients who turn to them.

You can view the following breast cancer videos online via DSL, Cable, T1 - 147Kbps:

- Introduction to Breast Cancer
- How Breast Cancer Spreads
- Factors that Affect Cure Rate
- Determining the Stage of Breast Cancer
- Chemotherapy and Hormone Therapy
- Radiation Therapy
- Brachytherapy and other new treatment options
- Patient Stories
- The Next Step - Deciding on a Treatment

http://cancer.sutterhealth.org/inf
ormation/bc_videos.html

About the Authors...

Cindy Daniel - Cindy is a research coordinator by day and a mystery writer by night. She is the author of the *Death Warmed Over Mystery Series,* featuring amateur sleuth Hannah Garrett. With two books in the series published, she is now hard at work on a new series called *Mad Moms In Minivans.*

Cindy lives in a lakeside suburb of Dallas, with her husband Jeff, three dogs, and a cat. She hopes to be a grandma some day soon!

Robin Cieszinski - Robin lives in Royse City, a suburb of Dallas, Texas, with her husband Mike and their two dogs. When she's not busy at work as an escrow officer, she is at home in the country watching sports, enjoying movies, or creating a new scrapbook; or trying to create a new Cieszinski.

Nancee Biank - Nancee Biank, MSW, LCSW, was the Director of Children and Family Services at

Wellness House, Hinsdale, Illinois, a nonprofit organization that offers psychosocial support to cancer patients and their families for over ten years. She developed the ground-breaking Family Matters Program for children who have a parent with cancer.

Nancee is the author of several chapters in various clinical books and journals, and is currently working on a book for families titled: *Tell Them That We Know...Children's Responses to Illness and Loss.*

Nancee is in private practice and is cofounder of Partners in Transition in Hinsdale, Illinois. She trained at the Institute for Psychoanalysis, Child and Adolescent Therapy Program, Chicago, Illinois, the University of Illinois, Jane Adams College of Social Work in Chicago, Illinois.

She lives with her husband, Vincent, in Hinsdale and enjoys spending time with her three young grandchildren.

Dont forget to visit our website!

Not My Mom!

A place where you can
share your thoughts, your fears,
and your stories of surviving

www.notmymom.com